EMOTION AND INSANITY

Founded by C. K. Ogden

The International Library of Psychology

ABNORMAL AND CLINICAL PSYCHOLOGY
In 19 Volumes

EMOTION AND INSANITY

S THALBITZER

Preface by Harald Höffding

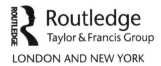
Routledge
Taylor & Francis Group

LONDON AND NEW YORK

First published in 1926 by
Kegan Paul, Trench, Trubner & Co., Ltd.
2 Park Square, Milton Park, Abingdon, Oxfordshire OX14 4RN
711 Third Avenue, New York, NY 10017

First issued in paperback 2014

Routledge is an imprint of the Taylor and Francis Group, an informa business

British Library Cataloguing in Publication Data
A CIP catalogue record for this book
is available from the British Library

Emotion and Insanity
ISBN 0415-20935-8
Abnormal and Clinical Psychology: 19 Volumes
ISBN 0415-21123-9
The International Library of Psychology: 204 Volumes
ISBN 0415-19132-7

ISBN 13: 978-1-138-87492-3 (pbk)
ISBN 13: 978-0-415-20935-9 (hbk)

CONTENTS

PREFACE

It is possible to have a very high opinion of Experimental Psychology without believing that it is the only way of approaching the Mind. In fact, only relatively elementary processes can be investigated by its means. The more developed and complicated the phenomena the more we must base ourselves on direct observation.

Signs are not wanting that Descriptive Psychology is once more coming to the front. Works like Alexander Shand's *Foundations of Character* (1914) and, previous to this, Heinrich Maier's *Psychologie des emotionalen Denkens* (1908) are indicative of such a tendency.

But in addition to works like these, based on the study of normal mental states there is another group which is of particular importance for descriptive psychology, namely those devoted to clinical psychiatry. If a psychiatrist is also gifted as a psychologist and is familiar with the cultural problems and historical forms of the higher mental life, he has this advantage over the " pure " psychologist, that his clinical experience provides him with a wealth of mental forms, which, though distorted and awry, yet by this very fact throw light on the

PREFACE

general psychical laws, especially where the normal
passes over into the abnormal through countless
intermediate stages. Clinical observation can be
more careful and fundamental than ordinary observation, where as a rule the subject-matter is presented only for a few brief moments. Moreover, the
psychiatrist can combine thorough-going physiological investigation with observations of a purely
psychological nature.

For my part I have profited greatly by the study
of psychiatry, and the basis of my psychological
position is due to my interest in this field. I am
therefore glad to find that the author of the work to
which I am contributing this Preface endeavours
to make the results of psychiatry available for
general psychological enquiry and emphasizes the
significance of psychiatric research for the understanding of normal mental processes. It is hardly
necessary to add that my interest in the work itself
is not due to the fact that the author adopts various
views that I myself have put forward. This need no
more prevent my introducing the work to a wider
public than the fact that on other points the author's
views differ from my own.

In two respects in particular the author has, I feel,
made important contributions to psychology. In
the first place there is the general conclusion at
which he has been enabled to arrive by a study of
the manic-depressive psychosis. He shows that
within this we find every kind of feeling represented
—even the most complicated—and on a more

PREFACE

elaborate scale, so that each particular feature appears with greater clearness. We thus become aware of features which are not easily discovered in the observation of normal processes.

Secondly there is his description and analysis of " mixed forms " at various levels, of those mental states in which different feeling-elements are in operation simultaneously and with opposite and contrasted effects, so that the elements are set off one against another. At the first level we have one such mixed form in " active productive melancholia," where deep unpleasure is combined with intensified motor unrest and great instability of thought. In higher forms the relations become continually more complicated, so that not only are pleasure and un-pleasure set off against one another but some definite mental content exercises an influence on the character of the feeling.

In dealing with such mixed forms the author might also have referred to the Danish psychologist Sibbern, who was the first clearly to describe such phenomena.

I need only add that there is one point on which I think I have perhaps been misunderstood by Thalbitzer. I do not regard Will as merely parallel to Thought and Feeling. I have used the term " willing " in the widest sense, as a generic term for urge, instinct (i.e. urge and capacity in immediate conjunction), impulse, wish, proposal, resolve. Will, in my view, is the foundation of all psychic life ; and it is to this foundation that we must relate

PREFACE

our analysis of thought and feeling in all its stages. It is only by way of preliminary explanation that at the beginning of my Psychology I describe the psyche as " that which thinks, feels, and wills." As the outcome of my investigations I might define it as " that which behaves thinkingly and feelingly." I am here more in agreement with the author than he supposes himself to be in agreement with me.

It would give me great satisfaction were the present work to find a public in other countries, and it has my best wishes as thus presented to English readers.

HARALD HÖFFDING

CARLSBERG, COPENHAGEN.

INTRODUCTION

A

CHAPTER I

INTRODUCTION

WHEN an oculist or a kidney-specialist opens a book on the physiology of the eye or the kidney, he will always, except in matters of detail, share the general views of the author as to the function and product of the organ under discussion ; for, as a rule, author and reader have the same premises. The point of view of each is based on the same broad foundation of general physiological training which they have acquired by their medical education and practice.

It is quite otherwise with the mental specialist, who hopes, by the study of a psychological work, to get some help towards the explanation of mental phenomena whether they are the result of a diseased or of a healthy brain. Only too often the mental specialist has the impression that between him and the psychological writer there yawns an impassable gulf. It is as if each were speaking a language of his own, incomprehensible to the other. They lack the common basis which is necessary for mutual understanding. As a

3

rule the mental specialist stands (and ought to stand firmly) on a foundation of general physiological knowledge which he has acquired through his medical training and his experience as a doctor and which has, as it were, become part of him ; the psychological writer, on the other hand, has usually quite different premises. The explanation is not difficult to find.

From early times mental phenomena have been the object of burning interest and fantastic speculation on the part of human beings. Ancient philosophers buried themselves in psychological studies and drew up wise systems and classifications ; and psychology had already made considerable progress when the beginnings of a really scientific physiology first appeared. Psychology, therefore, had a great advantage over this comparatively young science.

In the course of time, as it was gradually recognized that even mental phenomena correspond to the activity of a material organism, the human brain, psychologists certainly were not unwilling to take physiology into their service, but as a rule they did so only when its conclusions did not conflict with the prevailing psychological views of the time. In the latter event, psychology, by virtue of its seniority and its wide scope, exercised a tyranny in the province of cerebral physiology which cannot be said to have wholly disappeared even to-day. It is certainly now generally recognized that the brain, as an organ of the body, must be subject to the same main physiological laws as all other organs, and as a necessary consequence psychology must abandon its isolation and take its place as one branch of the physiology of the whole body. Yet physiological writers are constantly found approaching psychological questions (*i.e.* questions of brain physiology) with a nervous caution and uncertainty which is chiefly caused by the fear of taking a purely physiological view of the brain (*i.e.* of mental processes) and thereby offending current psychological opinion. As a rule physiologists prefer to avoid the subject, in order not to arouse the watchful jealousy of the psychologists, which allows no one who is regarded as an outsider to approach a province which they consider theirs and theirs alone, and in which they desire at all costs to maintain their supremacy.

About the middle of the last century, at a time when psychology seemed to have proceeded as far as was possible along the paths which it had hitherto followed, an attempt was made to open up a new avenue to the understanding of the activity of the human brain ; and thus arose the science called psycho-physics. Its object was to try to throw light on the operations of the human brain by measuring all the results of psychic activity which were regarded as capable of measurement. The direct and true descendant of this psycho-physics is the psycho-physiology of the present day.

The exponents of this science have in past years produced an immense literature and a vast store of material in the form of measurements of the functioning of the sense-organs, of associative processes, of the use of the muscles, of vaso-motor organic changes under varying conditions, etc. ; and in this way there has been produced much raw material, valuable in part perhaps and sometimes interesting, and recorded to some extent in curves and charts. Whether the gain corresponds in any measure to the time and labour involved may certainly be regarded as doubtful.

Of course it will always be interesting to record by means of charts and curves anything in this province that is measurable, but it must be remembered that only comparatively peripheral phenomena can be explained by this means, while the essence of the matter, namely, what happens in the central organ, will certainly remain for ever beyond the reach of mathematical treatment. Certain exponents of psycho-physiology have not realized this, and attempt, often by means of quite arbitrary interpretations of their for the most part highly ambiguous curves and charts, to arrive at far-reaching and quite untenable conclusions about the activity of the brain. Thus, insufficiently grounded in physiology and indifferent exponents of psychology as psycho-physiologists have unfortunately often proved themselves, they have brought their science into discredit among psychologists who think on physiological lines. They have often been so blindly devoted to their experiments and their curves, that they quite fail to notice if their results contradict the facts which lie plainly before them in daily life, or are at cross purposes with universal and established physiological truths.

But though we should not expect too much from modern psycho-physiology, there is another science closely related to psychology, the results of which, especially in the last few years, seem to have influenced psychology only in a small degree, but will certainly in the future form a very important source for it ; I refer to modern psycho-pathology or psychiatry, the science of mental diseases. Here and there in psychological work we certainly meet an attempt to use the practical knowledge of this science ; but as soon as psychologists venture on to psycho-pathological ground, they grope about as a rule in an amazingly dilettante fashion. This is not a reproach ; it is in itself quite intelligible. For modern psychiatry, even though a new science, has already covered so wide a range that it alone is sufficient to demand a man's complete service.

There is danger in the fact that the psychopathological conditions which have most strongly attracted the attention of psychological writers are the hysterical ones; for among mental diseases there is probably hardly any group which needs greater care and psychiatric experience in analysis than the hysterical, if we are not to be completely misled. While psychological writers cannot for the most part be considered competent to venture into the province of psychiatry and profit by its experiences, it cannot be maintained that the contrary holds good. It is true that as far as weight of erudition and extensive reading in the specifically psychological sphere are concerned, the psychiatrist cannot as a rule compete with the professional psychologist; but what he lacks in the way of theory he can make up to a very considerable extent by practice. It is the daily and constant duty of the mental specialist to penetrate into the mental life of human beings; he is in reality the practical psychologist *par excellence,* or at any rate he can find in his daily life the conditions under which he may become so. Moreover, the work of the mental specialist naturally leads him, even outside the hospital and the consulting room, to adopt almost involuntarily the same observant and scrutinizing attitude towards those whom he meets in ordinary life as he does every day towards his patients. And the knowledge and understanding of normal mental life is naturally just as important for the mental specialist as the knowledge of the activity of the healthy eye or the healthy kidney is for the oculist or the kidney-specialist. On the other hand, it will be obvious that the knowledge of various abnormal mental conditions can be of great value for the understanding of the corresponding normal states. That the knowledge of pathological states may often be profitably used to throw light on corresponding normal conditions is a point of view which is not new or surprising to doctors. We all know how deeply indebted our normal anatomy and physiology are to pathology, and this holds good not least of cerebral and neuro-pathology.

What should we know of many of the centres now definitely established in the cerebral cortex, or of their tracts to and from the periphery, had we not learnt to understand them by investigating cases of degeneration of those tracts, brought on by abnormal processes ? What should we know of the position of the various reflex tracts if they had not been established by the examination of pathological cases ? That it is possible similarly to profit by the study of certain kinds of mental diseases in order to arrive at an understanding of the corresponding normal mental conditions, I shall endeavour to show in the following pages.

Psychologists, then, far from being justified in refusing, as many of them do, to accept the conclusions of psychiatrists under the pretext that they understand *only* abnormal conditions, ought rather to look upon the psychiatrist's knowledge of abnormal conditions *also* as an advantage which he has over them. The psychologist who rejects the psychiatrist's contributions to the elucidation of psychological problems under the pretext that he understands only abnormal mental life is as false in his judgment as the anatomist or physiologist who denies to the oculist or kidney-specialist the right to join in the discussion of the normal structure and function of the organ in question. When I plead in the preceding paragraphs so strongly for the right of the psychiatrist to take a part, and even a very important one, in the discussion of psychological questions, it is not because psychological as well as psycho-physiological works have not already been written by psychiatrists ; but in almost all works of this kind with which I am acquainted the authors seem from the outset to be prejudiced in favour of the system and point of view of one or another psychological school. The moment they take pen in hand to treat of a psychological subject, they seem to lose sympathy with their original mother-science, and to forget the foundation acquired through their medical training in the knowledge of fundamental physiological laws which hold good wherever we find the functioning of the living organ.

Of far greater value for psychologically minded psychiatrists is the tendency within psychology to base itself, without being hoodwinked by psycho-physiology and its pseudo-exact method, on careful observation and close study of the diverse experiences of daily life. One of the most eminent living exponents of this Psychology of Experience is the Danish philosopher Höffding, to whose point of view I shall often refer in the following pages. Höffding's power of observation is usually so reliable and his view, especially of psychic phenomena, is so simple and close to life that it is doubtful whether any other psychological method can find such support in physiology. Without the physiological premises which can probably be given only by medical training, Höffding conceives psychical phenomena, their constitution and their history, in such a way that his conception of them involuntarily harmonizes in almost every detail with a physiological method of regarding the brain and its function. But while Höffding, in various points, still observes a certain caution in the conclusions which he draws from the almost complete parallelism between his psychological observation and a physiological conception of the activity of the brain, the present author aims at drawing the natural and necessary conclusions unhesitatingly and completely. And it will certainly prove possible in this way to reach a clearer understanding of human mental life in certain directions, especially those manifestations of it which we call moods, feelings and emotions.

PSYCHOLOGY

CHAPTER II

IT is to empirical psychology that we owe the familiar distinction between three different sides or elements in mental activity. In every psychical process, in every concrete mental product, we always find these three essentially different elements : intellectual activity, feeling and will. According to whether the first, second or third of these elements is the predominating one, the concrete psychical products are classed as intellectual processes, affective states and manifestations of will. A division into three mental elements is natural also in a consideration of the brain from the physiological point of view and is also confirmed by the findings of psycho-pathology.

A more thorough investigation of these circumstances considered in conjunction with certain pathological facts about the brain, will, however, as we shall presently see, necessitate a shifting of the dividing line which has hitherto been drawn by psychologists between elementary intellectual acti-

vity and that side of mental life which is
actively directed outwards.

A

Feeling is the psychical element which is
recognized as pleasure or displeasure (unpleasure) according to its positive or negative
direction. A more exact definition of these
opposites (pleasure and displeasure) cannot be
given, because feeling as a psychical element
cannot be further analysed or traced back to
anything simpler. It must suffice to indicate
the psychical processes in which feeling is the
predominating element and which we call
affective states.

These fall naturally into three groups:
moods, feelings and emotions. The dividing
line between these groups is uncertain; the
difference between them is chiefly a difference
of quantity and is based on differences in
intensity, suddenness and duration. Affective
states of comparatively little intensity which
begin slowly and die down gradually and yet
as a rule last for a considerable time, are
called Moods. Feelings are distinguished from
moods principally by their greater intensity;
and, lastly, Emotions are distinguished from
the preceding affective states by their sudden
appearance, their considerable intensity, their
comparatively short duration and rapid
cessation.

From this it is obvious that it is often a matter of opinion which of the three groups should include those affective states which lie between them. Further, the dividing lines between them are obliterated by the inaccuracy of ordinary speech and a lack of shades of expression; a word like gladness, for example, is used as often of an affective process as of a feeling or a mood. In any case, however, an exact division between these three types of affective states is unimportant for the present investigation.

Within the different groups of affective states each single process is characterized partly by the intellectual elements which it contains, partly by the impulses to movement and action which are included in it, but chiefly by the different way in which pleasure and displeasure mingle and conflict with one another in each single affective state.

As we shall see in what follows, it is only very seldom (if indeed ever in adult and developed individuals) that we find pure unmixed states of pleasure and displeasure. The higher the intellectual development of the individual, the more nuances and facets will there be as a rule in his feelings. This rich variety of shading in the element of feeling is, however, due entirely to the varying ways in which the opposites pleasure and displeasure combine and conflict with one another.

EMOTION AND INSANITY

Wilhelm Wundt, who was chiefly responsible for the present psycho-physiological school in Germany, and whose teaching held sway in German psychology for almost half a century, advances in his works * the theory that there are three dimensions of feeling. Besides the ' dimension ' pleasure-unpleasure, Wundt thinks that he can distinguish two other dimensions in which the psychical phenomenon of feeling can move—namely, the dimension of excitation and quiescence and the dimension of tension and relaxation ; and he tries to illustrate this idea by means of a drawing in which two of these dimensions are represented as two lines on the plane of the paper intersecting one another at right angles, while the third is imagined to run from front to back on a plane which cuts that of the paper vertically.

Now it is significant that Wundt in ascribing these three dimensions (or the ability to move in them) to the psychical phenomenon feeling, uses only a diagram, a comparison which he has taken from the external material world. This diagram by which Wundt seeks to illustrate his idea, has, however, the great fault that it cannot be imagined nor indeed can one form any notion of it. Only those things which appear in spatial form are or can be conceived to be of three dimensions.

* *Physiologische Psychologie*, 6th edition, I (1908), II (1910), and III (1911) ; also *Psychologie*, 11th edition (1913).

18

But to conceive of a psychical phenomenon in spatial form is an impossibility; it is not possible to imagine a spherical feeling or a pyramidal or cone-shaped affective process. Wundt's three-dimensional theory of feeling is based from the first on a completely false analogy.

Moreover, apart from the uselessness of this diagram of dimensions, a three-dimensional conception of a psychical phenomenon would be quite unphysiological. Feeling as a psychical phenomenon must correspond to cerebral activity, *i.e.* to the activity of the brain-cells; and these, like all other living cells, are governed by the law that under physiological conditions there can only be an increase or decrease of their specific function. A movement of the cell-function in several different dimensions is quite unknown to physiology.

Finally, it is not clear what Wundt means by the dimensions excitation-quiescence and tension-relaxation. No psychologist, and indeed no one who is at all interested in psychology, can be in any doubt as to the meaning of pleasure-unpleasure; but excitation and tension must be the excitation and tension of something. Wundt, however, leaves us in ignorance of what that 'something' may be; at times by excitation he seems to mean intellectual excitation (which may however be found in various affective states),

19

and by tension, psycho-motor tension ; with
corresponding meanings for quiescence and
relaxation. But whatever he may mean,
excitation-quiescence and tension-relaxation
are psychical phenomena which cannot by
any means be classed with pleasure-unpleasure
as forms or dimensions of the element feeling ;
on the contrary, as far as they are present,
they must (in spite of Wundt's energetic
protest) be thought of as organic sensations,
various organic sensations being indeed associ-
ated with almost all mental states.

When I defined affective states as the
psychical processes in which the feeling factor
predominates, I was not thinking solely or
chiefly of the intensity of that element.
The intensity of different elements is difficult
to compare or to measure. I had in mind
chiefly the degree in which the feeling is
characteristic of the state. We see writers on
psychology (for example, Höffding) classifying
phenomena like hunger, thirst or fatigue as
feelings. This is certainly unjustified. By
these states we mean, for the most part,
organic sensations in which the affective tone
may be greater or less, or different in different
circumstances ; and the most decisive factor
in this question seems to me to be that the
affective tone in itself plays only an unimportant part in characterizing the state. We
may have hunger with unpleasant or pleasant
tones (' pleasantly hungry '), and we may have

a sensation of hunger which to some extent is emotionally indifferent, such as the hunger which is felt at the customary meal-times. But in all these cases it is hunger without reference to the affective tone, which must therefore be regarded as something quite irrelevant as far as the hunger is concerned. The same is true of fatigue and thirst; they are not affective states, because their affective tone plays an unimportant part in their characterization; their chief characteristic is the collection of organic sensations of which they are composed, which we all know and which may have varying affective tones according to circumstances.

A physiological method of observing the affective states, such as is used in the following pages, must, of course, aim at dividing or grouping them according to their physiological constitution; but various psychological writers (even those who call themselves psycho-physiologists) attempt to group feelings as autopathic, sympathetic, æsthetic, ethical, religious, etc.

It is difficult to see how such a classification of feelings according to their *intellectual* content, a classification which might be continued *ad infinitum*, can have any special value for the psychology of *feelings*. It is, of course, quite useless for a physiological consideration and classification of affective states. Feeling is feeling, whether it is pleasure or displeasure

or varying compounds of these opposites ;
and this is true irrespective of whether the
intellectual processes to which the feeling is
attached are of a religious, æsthetic, ethical
or other nature.

B

The basis of all intellectual activity is
sensation. Human consciousness receives
sensations through the eye and the ear,
through the senses of taste and smell and
through the various organs of sense in the
skin ; sensations also reach the brain from the
mucous membranes, muscles and joints, from
the intestines and glands, and indeed from
all interior organs.

All these sensations are the bed-rock on
which the whole intellectual side of mental
life rests, the necessary presuppositions for all
ideas and thoughts. Of the sensations we
need here to discuss in detail only that of
pain, because there is a certain confusion of
thought on this point among various physiological as well as psychological writers, and
this confusion also affects the province of the
feeling-element. It is due to some extent to
the lack of clearness in poetic and also in
daily speech, so that the word pain is used in
the same sense as displeasure without its
being made clear that in this case it is a
question of metaphor, a poetic analogy, a com-

parison, which has been taken from another psychic sphere.

We often speak in a figurative sense of ' mental ' pain under conditions of strong displeasure which have nothing to do with ' bodily ' pain, *i.e.* the sensation of pain which arises for example through lesion of the skin or in processes of irritation or inflammation of internal and external organs. But unfortunately it is not always clear that we are here concerned with a metaphor, though we are familiar enough with the use of similar metaphors derived from the different senses. We speak of the sweetness of love, of dark thoughts, of a cold tone, of noisome self-praise or of warm interest, without anyone seriously attributing to these phenomena any influence on our senses of taste or smell, on our eyes or on our organs for sensing temperature. The justification for the use of such metaphorical language must naturally lie in a certain similarity of feeling-tone between the two compared phenomena. But it is unfortunately not always so clearly realized that there is a completely similar connection and that we are speaking only in metaphor by means of a descriptive analogy when we talk of a painful loss or a mental pain.

A physiologist like Tigerstedt remarks that it is very difficult to draw a line between true pain (such as toothache or the pains of birth) and the feeling of displeasure ; and even a

psychologist such as Höffding has not succeeded in keeping apart the feeling of displeasure and the sensation of pain. This is
especially inconvenient in the first section of
Chapter VI in his Psychology, where Höffding
is discussing feeling. He there speaks several
times of the feeling of pain and throughout
uses the terms pain and displeasure of the
same psychic phenomenon. He thereby more
than once causes confusion and misunder-
standing partly in his interpretation of certain
observations made under normal conditions,
partly in his treatment of the pathological
phenomenon of analgesia (insensitivity to
pain), although this very phenomenon ought
to have led him on to the track of the correct
connection. He even mentions that the
severance of the grey substance of the spinal
marrow causes analgesia in the lower part of
the body ; but it can hardly be Höffding's
meaning that the elementary psychic phenomenon of the unpleasure-feeling is caused by
this grey substance of the spinal marrow.

That it has been possible for this confusion
between pain and displeasure to arise, is due,
of course, to the fact that in the majority of
cases the sensation of pain has a displeasure-
tone. To define pain as a sensation accompanied by strong displeasure is, however,
quite insufficient, partly because sensations in
almost all the fields of sense may have a
displeasure-tone (for example, a bad taste or

smell, false tones, cold feet, etc.) without having any connection with pain, and partly because we know of sensations of pain which have absolutely no displeasure-tone and may even to a greater or less degree have a pleasure-tone.

Pain-sensations may often be emotionally quite indifferent ; or greater pain-sensations may become so through repetition, if one is prepared for them or has grown accustomed to them ; and this may happen without the pain-sensation having decreased to any considerable extent. Even strong sensations of pain may appear in certain circumstances with a great sensation of pleasure. A colleague whose gift of observation I have often had occasion to verify, has told me, for example, that toothache often has for him a pleasure-tone, especially that painful throbbing which every one has experienced in toothache ; and he declares that this pleasure-tone has not the least connection with other ideas, but is connected entirely with the toothache. The same colleague has also observed a similar case in his practice ; a lady with a whitlow said that it certainly was painful but that the intermittent painful throbbing in the inflamed finger was accompanied by a quite definite feeling of pleasure ; this lady was therefore able quite unconsciously to distinguish between the sensation of pain and its feeling-tone.

On the whole I believe that anyone who is still prejudiced by having had popular views on this question instilled into him, will discover by careful observation that pain with a pleasure-tone is a by no means infrequent phenomenon and that the psychology of women in particular frequently affords examples of it. Probably this is especially true of female sexual psychology.

It follows from the preceding remarks that it must be equally reprehensible in scientific psychological terminology to speak of a *feeling* of pain or of a *feeling* of cold or of a *feeling* of touch. Pain, like cold or touch, is a sensation, of which the peripheral organs are in the skin, the mucous membrane and the internal organs, whence impressions are transferred by centripetal nerves to the sensory roots of the spinal nerve and thence through the lateral columns of the spinal nerve (probably in the Gower fasciculus), intersecting one another, to the different centres of the cerebral cortex (probably to its ascending parietal convolution).

After this digression we return to our starting-point, the intellectual side of mental life ; this includes all sensation and all thought. It now appears that it is possible only by abstraction to draw a clear line between sensation and thought. More exact analysis shows that even the simplest sensation presupposes memory, differentiation and comparison, and proves itself therefore to be elementary thought (Höffding) ; sensation and thought may therefore be treated under one heading.

The active element in all intellectual activity is, as Höffding emphasizes, of the greatest importance for the physiological understanding of the intellectual side of mental life. There is no such thing as a completely passive sensation. "At no point are we completely receptive" (Höffding). In order that a sensation may arise, there is need not only of a stimulus, of an impression from the outside world, but also of a certain activity, of a movement towards the impression or a readiness for it, without which no sensation at all can arise.

From daily experience we know that of the infinite number of impressions which we encounter in the course of the day, the majority arouse no sensation at all, others arouse a weak, indistinct, transitory sensation ; while the few impressions for which our brain-cells are ready and towards which they are addressed, or which by their strength or unwontedness attract to themselves the activity of the brain-cells, give the clear concise sensations.

Analogous to this is the fact that there is no completely passive thought ; "we never are completely passive in our association of ideas any more than we are passive in sensation " (Höffding). There is always a kind of choice or preference among the possible ideas, even where we try to follow the current of our thoughts while we are really guiding it. It is this active character of all sensation which we call attention, and it is the most elementary form of the will, while the active character of thought, which is recognizable as choice or preference, is the phenomenon which we call the inner will in the narrower sense.

As higher forms of intellectual activity are reached, its active side develops much more highly and may finally appear as that highly developed form which we find in logical thought. " We can thus prove a gradual ascent from unconscious to conscious but involuntary activity and thence to voluntary activity and true volition " (Höffding). The difference between the attention which is simple observation and the most highly developed will which is recognizable as choice, preference and determination, is therefore only a difference of degree. " There is a volition, an active side to each state of consciousness. There is only a difference of degree between our state during the forming of a decision and other states," says Höffding ; and he adds later : " the phenomena of will which are specially so called denote only the culminating points of a process which extends over the whole conscious life."

Höffding's constant and strong emphasis on the active character of the intellectual side of mental life arose probably in the first instance from his thorough psychological observations and reflections, but at the same time Höffding certainly sees clearly that it coincides exactly with a physiological view of the same conditions ; for, referring to Verworn, he writes in his Psychology : " Each organic being, apart from outside influence, is purely spontaneous in any given activity, and influences from without can produce only changes in that activity and nothing absolutely new."

This spontaneous activity of living organs which as far as the brain is concerned appears as a readiness of the brain-cells to receive impressions and is the physiological correlate of the psychic phenomenon of attention, the most elementary form of will — this spontaneous activity of the organs is the phenomenon which in physiology is called the tonus of the organs. Every living cell, including those of the brain, has an intrinsic tone, *i.e.* it shows at all times a certain degree of its specific activity ; a living cell never stands still like a machine which is stopped ; the difference between what happens in a ' working ' and in a ' resting ' cell is only a difference of degree and of intensity. And the tonus of the brain - cells of sensation and thought is therefore the physiological correlate of the whole human life of volition.

EMOTION AND INSANITY

By others, even by Höffding, the will is
usually regarded as a psychical element which
differs from feeling and conception and is an
adjunct to them. In accordance with the
argument developed in the preceding paragraphs, this cannot be admitted if we take
a physiological view-point. Will, that is,
activity, is not a psychical element differing
from perception and thought ; but thought
and will are two inseparable sides of the same
psychical element. It is impossible to imagine
them separated.

Although nothing prevents us from thinking in abstract terms of intellectual activity
without a feeling-tone or of feeling without
intellectual activity, a similar abstract method
of considering thought and will is impossible ;
if one is removed, the other immediately disappears. It is not possible to will without
the help of thoughts and it is equally impossible to think without that activity (*i.e.* the
Will) which is the expression for the tonus of
the cells of sensation and thought. The
expression ' intellectual activity ' involves
will, for activity is the same as action or
movement and therefore as will. Such a point
of view by no means involves a degradation
or depreciation of the status of the will in
mental life but rather assigns to the will a
more original and important position than
that which falls to the psychical elements.

Although Höffding strongly emphasizes the

position of the will as an independent psychical element, he gives it, nevertheless, a certain special status when he says : " If one of the three types of the elements of consciousness is to be considered the fundamental form of conscious life, it would have to be the will. Activity is a fundamental characteristic of the life of our consciousness." And when he later describes the will as " the true basis of mental life " and closes his chapter on the psychology of the will with the following sentence : " The will has a *still greater claim* than cognition and feeling, to be called an element, *i.e.* an original side or quality of mental life," it seems to me that Höffding by the words " still greater claim," which I have emphasized, supports my view that the will cannot be placed *by the side* of feeling and cognition.

C

In general, then, the will is classed by psychologists as the third mental element. This element has, however, always caused much puzzling and discussion, and not un-justifiably so. Above all, the will has a property which is very dangerous in an element, namely that it may be further resolved into two phenomena, the inner and the outer will ; this fact alone is sufficient to give us pause. The outer will manifests itself, according to the general view, by means

31

of movement or action. If, however, we examine the inner will more closely, we find in it exactly the same things which we found in all thought, *i.e.* ideas based on activity, and association of ideas. The inner will and thought are in reality identical phenomena and are not two fundamentally different elements in juxtaposition. At the moment when we pass from intellectual activity to movement and action, for the first time a new third psychical element is introduced, *psycho-motor innervation*, the impulse to movement and action which proceeds from the motor-centres of the brain. I can imagine that some may hesitate to recognize psycho-motor innervation as a *psychical* element, but this hesitation must soon disappear in the case of anyone who looks on the grey matter of the cerebral cortex as the material correlative of the human mind ; and surely we all do that.

Psycho-motor innervation possesses, besides the different sensory qualities, the indisputable advantage above all other elementary psychic activities, that we can confidently locate it in the cerebral cortex, in the ascending frontal convolution of the brain. The fact that we were able to locate the sensory centres and the psycho-motor centre of the brain earlier than the centres for the other elementary mental functions, arises naturally from the fact that these two activities of sensation and motor innervation are the two sides of mental life which are directed towards our environment. They correspond to one another like consignor and consignee. Their position with regard to one another is, as it were, symmetrical, as the centres of the sense organs are the first and the psycho-motor centres the last station by which the brain and the outside world communicate with one another ; they are the entrance and exit doors for all that affects the human mind. " As the psychology of cognition begins with sensation, so the psychology of will ends with the impulse to movement " (Höffding).

A special indication of the small degree to which psychology has understood how to profit by advances in the physiology and pathology of the brain, is given in my opinion by the fact that Fritsch and Hitzig's epoch-making discovery of the psycho-motor centres and their localization in the ascending frontal convolution, has, as it were, passed without leaving a trace over the opinions of psycho-logists about the psychology of the will. This discovery could and should have opened their eyes to the fact that psycho-motor innervation is an elementary psychical func-tion which represents the active side of the mind, and that the will, which had hitherto been regarded as a psychical element (albeit a somewhat troublesome one), really is a con-

E

glomeration, an artificial combination of psycho-motor innervation with what has been called ' inner will ' and is therefore identical with all thought.

In exact agreement with the view set forth above of the motor-active side of mental life as a psychical element, we have also the analytical treatment given by the modern psychiatric clinic to the different types within the group of mental diseases of mood, the manic-depressive psychosis. In the clinical treatment of this group of diseases we do actually distinguish between the changes which are seen in the spheres of intellectual life and of feeling and the changes in the psycho-motor sphere, a distinction which is especially necessary if we are to disentangle those aspects of the disease which are often difficult to understand without something of the kind and which we call the manic-depressive mixed types.

The outcome of this chapter can be summed up shortly as follows : A more exact psychological examination together with what is taught by modern cerebral physiology and psychiatry, must lead to a shifting of the hitherto universally accepted boundary between the intellectual and the active elements in mental life, so that the current division into the psychical elements of thought, feeling and will must be replaced by a classi-

PSYCHOLOGY
fication into intellectual activity, feeling and
psycho-motor innervation, and the mind may
briefly be defined, not as that which thinks,
feels and wills, but as that which thinks,
feels and acts.

An obvious proof of the extent to which
the will in its previous form has presented
difficulties to psychologists, is seen for example
in Wundt's treatment of the psychology of
the will.
Wundt treats the will-process as a special
class of affect and distinguishes between outer
and inner actions of the will according to
whether the process finds an outward expression by movement and action or not. Later
he lays it down that an affect is a necessary
presupposition for volitional action and each
volitional process is an emotion. Now there
can be no doubt that as a rule movement and
action are found as component parts of the
affect, that they find expression and comple-
tion (as the phrase is) by movements and
actions ; but there is no need on that account
to generalize and to maintain that every
volitional action presupposes an affect. Daily
life provides many examples where this is not
the case. For example, it would be impossible
for me to prove that any affect is presupposed
by the series of volitional actions which I go
through in dressing in the morning, tying my
tie, fastening my boots, going into the break-
35

fast-room, drinking coffee, lighting a cigar, looking at the morning paper, knocking the ash from my cigar, folding my paper and putting it away, etc. Life would be truly unbearable if in order to perform these and many other actions of the will, we had to pass from one affect to another.

Beside the above actions of the will and partly as their cause, there is certainly a number of intellectual processes which have usually a very weak feeling-tone. But if we are to call these ' affects ', as Wundt does, that would so extend the idea and the word ' affect ' that its meaning would be obliterated and it would become useless both in ordinary and in scientific language. The word ' affect ' is generally used almost in the same sense as ' emotion '—even emotions of great violence and intensity.

PSYCHIATRY AND PSYCHOLOGY

CHAPTER III

AN analysis of states of feeling such as will be attempted in this chapter presents various difficulties. Some of them are chiefly of a formal nature and are caused partly by the carelessness of daily and unfortunately often also of scientific language and partly by a certain poverty of language which does not keep pace with the diversity of life. We are too often obliged to group under the same terminology mental states which, although related, exhibit great psychological differences whether observed in others or in oneself, and at the same time differ in the physiological conditions for which they are the psychical expression.

It is a matter of daily experience, for example, not only that different people are glad in quite different ways but that in speaking of the same individual we use an expression like gladness for mental states which present aspects differing greatly from one another and therefore necessarily having correspondingly different physiological bases.

39

EMOTION AND INSANITY

More important than these more formal difficulties is the fact that the different moods, feelings, and emotions of human beings at their present stage of civilization are very often modified and changed by circumstances which do not concern the mental states themselves. Self-control is supposed to be one of the advantages of civilized man ; for the psychologist, however, it often causes such changes in the outward expression of many mental states, especially in the expression of states of feeling, that they become very unreliable as objects for his analysis. It might be expected that we should find states of feeling in their original and uninfluenced form among primitive peoples rather than in civilized races ; there are, however, not many of the former left ; and in any case there is not always an opportunity for studying them psychologically. The emotional life of children is more accessible for observation and study ; and this has therefore contributed substantially to the investigation of the psychology of emotional life and will continue to do so. But finally there is an immense material, probably the richest, for the elucidation of the psychology and physiology of the feeling-processes, which hitherto has hardly been worked up or used for this purpose, although some psychologists may have realized its importance in this respect. I refer to mental diseases, or to be more exact, to that

40

group of mental diseases which is called by modern psychiatry ' disorders of mood.' It is this rich material which will provide in this present work the principal means of elucidating the questions with which we are concerned.

The fact that the disorders of mood have hitherto not been much used to throw light on normal emotional life is due to a great extent to the relatively new classification of the mood-psychoses as an independent, clearly defined group of diseases. This does not mean that the great changes in emotional life which appear in almost all forms of mental disease, had hitherto been overlooked ; but the dividing line had not been clearly and consciously drawn between the mental diseases in which the abnormal mood for the main part is secondary in relation to the primary changes in the intellectual sphere (hallucinations and illusions), and the mental disorders in which the distortion of mood in one direction or the other is the essential factor.

The latter group, the genuine disorders of mood, is identical with the group of diseases which the greatest psychiatric systematizer of the present day, Kraepelin, classifies as manic-depressive insanity, in accordance with the delimitation which he adopted as a result of my work * and that of Dreyfus,† the term

* " The Manic-depressive Psychosis," 1902, and " Melancholy and Depression " in the *Allg. Zeitschrift für Psychiatrie und Nervenkrankheiten*, 1905.
† *Die Melancholie*, 1906.

having been originally introduced by him in 1899. The group covers those mental disorders which must be regarded as abnormal exaggerations of normal moods and feelings. When I define mood-psychoses as feelings exaggerated to an abnormal degree, that does not mean that these need in themselves be very strong ; pathological exaggeration may be expressed as well in the duration of the disease as in the violence of the symptoms. Even very strong moods and feelings in themselves are not necessarily diseased if they stand in only a transitory relationship to their cause, are an adequate reaction to it and die down after a duration of suitable length according to general human conditions. We may on the other hand find distorted moods which are much less intense than normal feelings, moods or emotions which an expert psychiatrist will not hesitate to call pathological because their duration is quite disproportionate to their cause (if indeed one is to be found). This very fact that the criterion for drawing the dividing line between the normal and the abnormal does not lie in the clinical type or the mood-type in itself, but in purely outward circumstances, i.e. the intensity or duration of the distorted mood in relationship to its cause, shows clearly the essential unity of the disorders of mood with our normal feelings and moods and their direct origin in the latter. Moreover, common to both normal and abnormal changes in mood is their ability to die down easily and quickly so that the individual returns to his healthy normal state of equilibrium. This characteristic of true mood-psychoses, that when they cease they leave no defect behind, plays a very important part in psychiatry because it is one of the principal points in which they differ from those forms of mental disease which, because of the strong secondary mood-changes which appear in them, may be often difficult enough to distinguish from true mood-psychoses and yet are based on profound qualitative changes, destructive processes in the cerebral cortex and its cells, processes which always leave a more or less clearly marked defect.

I regard patients who suffer from manic-depressive psychoses as the best material for the study of normal processes of feeling, and my reason for doing so can be clearly stated. To some extent there may be found within this group of diseases representatives of all, even the most complicated feelings, moods and emotions, and they appear usually with strongly defined lines and on a magnified scale ; we see them as if under the microscope with each characteristic feature standing out in bold relief ; we can observe the mood-psychosis as a natural mood or feeling raised, as it were, to a higher power. By this means it is often possible to obtain an insight

43

into those characteristics of the condition
which are less obvious or perhaps not even
noticeable in its normal dimensions. Also
there is as a rule in disorders of mood a complete disappearance of that factor which is
most disturbing to psychological investigation of the moods and feelings of the mentally
healthy civilized human being, *i.e.* self-control
and all the hindrances and modifications
which it causes. In the case of a patient
suffering from a mood-psychosis the state of
feeling usually develops unhindered in its
full strength and vigour ; it is chiefly on this
account that it is considered pathological.

Before we proceed to describe and analyse
the different forms of manic-depressive
psychosis and the physiological feelings and
moods which correspond to it, it must be made
clear that an analysis and description of this
kind necessitates a certain classification and
division under headings. Prototypes must be
set up which appear in their purely schematic
form perhaps seldom or never in real life, so
that they may serve as nuclei round which
the several infinitely varying conditions may
be naturally grouped. Schematization of this
kind is of course fully justified by its great
theoretical importance and is in reality very
necessary for the understanding of the whole
question. It must further be remembered
that when we speak in the following chapters
of mental *states* and *types* of disease, we are

44

making use of an abstraction. Since we are discussing a living organ, the brain, and its activity, there can be no question of states, but of processes ; we never have before us a state, something which remains or stands still, but always a process, something which advances, changing and altering continually. For this reason it may happen that in our analysis things may be regarded and described as simultaneous which really follow and replace one another. If this is clear, there can of course be no objection to describing and treating processes as if they were states in order to simplify analysis and make a general survey easier.

The manic-depressive psychosis or, as one ought perhaps more logically to call it, manic-melancholia has taken its name from the two types which are the extremes within this group and include all other forms of the disease.

By melancholia is understood scientifically and popularly sadness exaggerated to a diseased extent. The word Mania has been much misused in earlier psychology, especially at the time when the now forsaken doctrine of isolated psychical defects or monomanias was popular. This misuse has left its mark on ordinary speech, and people still speak of a ' mania ' for this or that. Scientifically, however, it has now been agreed that the word Mania should be used exclusively as a term for the mood of exaltation exaggerated to an abnormal extent, or pathological joy ; and thus it forms the exact opposite of melancholia or pathological sadness. The most obvious and characteristic fact in melancholia and in mania in their standard form is the change which appears in them in the emotional sphere, in the psychic element of feeling. Mania is marked by strongly exalted feeling or pleasure, and melancholia by deep unpleasure. Besides these changes in the emotional element of the two states it has however long been observed that corresponding changes appear in the intellectual and psycho-motor sphere ; and writers in early times already knew and described these. In typical melancholia there is found besides the intense feeling of displeasure a more or less obvious passivity, a slackness of all transversely striated muscles, which is recognizable in the physiognomy as well as in the carriage of the whole body ; in more advanced states the passivity takes the form of motor inhibition ; even the most vigorous challenge often is not able to arouse such inhibited patients to any active movement. These phenomena are caused chiefly by diminished innervation of the psycho-motor centres in the ascending frontal convolution of the brain. Beside these very obvious symptoms in feeling and psycho-motor activity, a more careful examination will find in melancholia corresponding changes

46

in the intellectual sphere, *i.e.* greatly decreased attention and therefore a more or less marked vacancy of mind.

We can therefore say that typical melancholia is passive and unproductive (*Melancholia passiva, improductiva*), the adjective passive referring to the psycho-motor side and unproductive to the intellectual side of this abnormal type, while the noun melancholia refers only to the deep depression, the change in the element of feeling.

All writers describe typical mania as the diametrical opposite of passive unproductive melancholia. Beside the highly exalted mood, the strongly marked feeling of pleasure, mania is characterized by an increased impulse toward movement ; the movements of the maniac are livelier, quicker and also more frequent and stronger than those of the normal human being, all this being the expression of the increased activity of his psycho-motor centres. This applies also to his speech ; the maniac talks incessantly, and this gives scope to his greatly increased intellectual productivity which, together with an alert and very easily distracted attention, forms the third main symptom of his disease, intellectual over-activity. Every mental specialist knows such patients ; they are boisterous and high-spirited, always moving and wandering about ; they interfere in everything, chatter, go from one object to another, and pay attention to everything within sight or earshot ; they can be caustic, witty, charming, or coarse ; their whole intellectual activity is characterized by what in technical language is called the ' flight of ideas.' Analogous to melancholia, we can therefore assign the adjectives active and productive to mania in its standard form (*Mania activa productiva*).

From observation of daily life and from introspection, we are all aware of moods which weakly reflect in each feature the two standard types of disease which have been outlined above—active productive mania and passive unproductive melancholia. Reducing these two psychoses to physiological dimensions and taking as it were their square root, we recognize the two natural moods or feelings of active talkative joy and quiet silent sadness.

From very early times mental specialists have noticed that by no means all cases of mania and melancholia correspond to the standard type, but that they may differ from them in one way or another. Formerly the classification of such cases often caused difficulty ; their place in the system was not clearly understood. Kraepelin was the first to give us the clue to the understanding of these variant forms, by demonstrating the existence of the manic-depressive (or manic-melancholic) complex types and indicating their place in the system. In the sixth edition of his Psychiatry, the first edition in which he classes manic-depressive psychosis as one single disease, Kraepelin calls attention to the fact that cases of mania are sometimes found which, far from exhibiting the increased activity characteristic of mania, give evidence on the contrary of obvious psycho-motor inhibition, a symptom usually attaching to melancholia ; and on the other hand we meet with cases of melancholia in which the customary motor inhibition is replaced by its opposite, a strong psycho-motor excitation which otherwise is found as a symptom of typical mania.

In a work published in the same year (1899) on The complex Conditions of Manic-depressive Insanity, Kraepelin's disciple Weygandt proved that on the intellectual side of mental life there may be a corresponding complexity. There are manias without flight of ideas and even with intellectual inhibition ; and on the other hand we find productive melancholics whose activity of mind is exactly like the flight of ideas which is characteristic of typical mania.

These clinical observations led to the classification of the manic-depressive complex types into all the varying forms into which this group was afterwards divided by Kraepelin in the later editions of his Psychiatry, and by me.* In addition to passive unproductive melancholia and active productive mania (the two limiting forms) we can from a purely schematic point of view reckon as possible types within the manic-depressive psychosis the six following manic-depressive complex forms :

Active unproductive melancholia
    ,,   productive   ,,
Passive   ,,   ,,

and

Passive productive mania
    ,,   unproductive ,,
Active   ,,   ,,

I call these six types complex types of the first order ; and it will be shown in the following pages that all these complex types of the disorders of mood have their corresponding normal feelings or moods.

The most characteristic and perhaps the most instructive complex form of the first order in mania-melancholia is active productive melancholia, earlier known by psychiatrists as agitated melancholia or anxiety-melancholia and often grouped separately in clinical classification. Active productive melancholia is characterized by the following symptoms or changes in the three chief mental spheres : deep unpleasure, greatly increased psycho-motor activity and a more

* *Den manio-depressive Psykose* (1902). Translated in op. cit., *Archiv für Psychiatrie,* 1908.

or less definite flight of ideas. Every mental
specialist knows this form of the disease ; the
patient with agitated melancholia suffers from
extreme unpleasure and a ceaseless motor
unrest which seldom allows him to remain
in bed, where he ought to be, but drives him
out on to the floor without repose, complain-
ing and wringing his hands ; everything that
comes within reach is made to share in his
restlessness ; the room of a patient suffering
in this way is often a model for the destruction
of Jerusalem.* Besides these symptoms we
see a more or less definite flight of ideas which
in many cases equals that found in productive
mania and shows itself in jerky chaotic lamen-
tations about all past, present and future mis-
fortunes and misery, for which the patient
more or less blames himself ; increased intellectual activity is also seen in his easily distracted and inconsequent thought ; every new
sense-impression, even the least important,
can attract his anxious attention.

If we reduce this exaggerated type of disease
to physiological dimensions, we recognize the
feeling and emotion which, in a man who is
mentally normal, is called anxiety. Its
psychic constituents are unpleasure, increased
motor activity and a more or less increased

* In the third chapter of my work mentioned above, a more
detailed account of each of the different forms of this mental
disease may be found. As part of these descriptions is in the
form of question and answer, I have succeeded in giving them a
certain dramatic vividness.

activity of mind. If the strength of these single elements is further reduced, we have the mood called worry (a weakened form of anxiety).

From observation and from introspection we also know forms which have the outward characteristics, anxiety, displeasure, and agitation, but in which flight of ideas is lacking or has changed into its opposite, intellectual inhibition. This feeling corresponds to the pathological complex form of active unproductive melancholia. This, of course, is not quite the same type as the productive, and has also not quite the same physiological or pathological basis ; yet we may correctly speak of this feeling also as anxiety, because it is hardly to be expected that speech should provide a special term for each of these outwardly similar feelings even if a more thorough psychological analysis shows a certain difference between them in the intellectual sphere.

The counterpart in psychiatric diagnosis to agitated melancholia is found in passive or inhibited mania (which in its extreme form is stuporose mania, called by Kraepelin originally, but not quite logically, manic stupor). The inhibited maniac lies or sits quietly, looking roguish and beamingly happy ; his feelings are much exalted while there is a decided inhibition of all movement. If motor inhibition is extended also to the muscles of the face, the strong feeling of pleasure may no longer appear directly in his features, or at most as a sort of cunning ; but as soon as we busy ourselves with the patient and are fortunate enough to overcome this inhibition, his mood betrays itself very soon in a beaming smile. As in agitated melancholia, so also in passive mania, intellectual activity may appear in various ways ; it may be either inhibited or decreased like the psycho-motor activity or exalted like the element of feeling. If mental activity is increased and volatile as in typical mania and if at the same time there is inhibition of the brain-centre of the speech mechanism,* we can observe a very curious phenomenon, in that the inhibited maniac after overcoming his speech-inhibition with immense effort in response to a vigorous challenge from the doctor, suddenly with a mischievous look utters a more or less vulgar joke or some biting piece of sarcasm and then immediately sinks back into his former blissful passivity or inhibition.

For example, I have for a number of years observed a well-educated lady, who, if I am successful in extracting an answer from her in her inhibited manic phases, utters explosively a couple of sharp words in loudly intoned

* The speech-centre (Broca's centre) in the third left frontal convolution has in the manic-depressive complex forms a certain independence in relation to the other psycho-motor centres ; its behaviour sometimes follows these and sometimes is opposed to them and may, for example, follow the mental activity in the direction of excitation or inhibition.

EMOTION AND INSANITY

French or English (she is a native of Copenhagen) with a very lively facial expression, and then sinks quickly into her former inhibited state of happiness. I therefore presumed that in her case there was a not inconsiderable flight of ideas which was unrecognizable only because motor inhibition had affected the speech-centre also ; and I was confirmed in this supposition when I questioned her in her relatively sane and only slightly exalted periods.

If, on the other hand, mental activity is also inhibited, we should have no other result from our efforts than the same quiet languishing smile or slight laugh. I have found also this last type, passive unproductive mania, excellently illustrated by one of my female patients. When I enter her room, she lies as a rule in bed rolled up in a ball and completely covered by the bed-clothes. If I draw the clothes from her face, I find her half-stifled with laughter which now becomes heartier or noisier ; but she does not speak a word even when spoken to, and she very seldom moves from her position ; occasionally, at most, she makes a gentle tired movement of the arm in my direction. In a regular, characteristic mania such an exuberant and unadulterated feeling of pleasure as hers would result in a torrent of words and a motor activity which would not allow her to stay in bed but would make her get up and dance.

54

The passive mania described above (whether productive or unproductive) is a form of disorder of mood with which every modern mental specialist is familiar and which he can classify correctly ; but at times it was a hard nut for our predecessors to crack. They often did not in the least understand this mania which seemed not to be real mania because it lacked the activity and mental volatility of typical mania ; these two symptoms seemed on the contrary to be replaced by the intellectual and motor inhibition which usually characterize melancholia.

As a matter of fact Kraepelin, and after him Weygandt, in their works on complex manic-depressive forms, were the first to lead the way to an understanding of these types which are often extremely strange.

The normal mood corresponding to passive mania is quiet joy, peaceful happiness. We all know people who keep remarkably quiet in a gay and noisy assembly, even though they may look very happy ; but sometimes such a person, after being a silent spectator for a long time, will suddenly surprise the rest of the company with a humorous, amusing or pointed remark that perhaps increases the noisy gaiety of the others while its author looks on with a quiet smile. In these cases we must assume that there is a certain inhibition or at any rate a comparative retardation of motor activity and perhaps also of intellectual productivity compared with what

55

is usually found with a similar feeling of pleasure and in the type seen in the rest of the laughing, chattering, noisy throng.

It will have been noticed in the types described above that inhibition or excitation of intellectual activity is not always easy to judge because it cannot always be directly observed by the investigator. In cases where psycho-motor inhibition affects the speech-centre, we are to some extent prevented from forming any definite opinion as to what and how the patients in question are thinking. Before we can know anything definite on this point, we usually have to await the moment when the patient's verbo-motor inhibition is removed or the illness is over. The manic-melancholic psychosis is as a matter of fact specially characterized by its periodic course and its completely or partially lucid intervals between the attacks; if during these the patient is questioned as to what was happening in him during the attack, very interesting facts may often be brought to light. In a case of this kind it may perhaps appear that a patient whose illness seemed to the investigator to be a form of typical, *i.e.* of inhibited or unproductive melancholia, in reality was suffering from a complex type, the fifth in the list, namely, a motor-inhibited but intellectually productive melancholia. This type is certainly far more frequent than is generally assumed; but productivity cannot always be detected because motor inhibition affects the speech-movements. Although it was not possible during the attack to make the patient utter even a syllable, he may be able in a lucid interval to tell of a number of depressive thoughts which occupied his mind during the abnormal period and which were concerned with past, present and future matters in the form of self-reproach and fear of present and future misfortune, with such intensity that they assumed the form of hallucinations, reproachful and threatening voices, the voice of conscience, God or the devil. These patients may at times surprise their doctor unpleasantly because it may afterwards appear that they have understood clearly and remember what has happened and has been said in their presence. In the belief that the strongly inhibited patient is taking no notice of what is said about him, an inexperienced psychiatrist may possibly make some careless remark, and it may be rather painful to him to be reminded of it later by the patient.

At times the flow of thought of an inhibited but productive melancholic may be able to turn so hastily from one painful subject to another that the patient has a right to some extent to talk of 'inner' anxiety, in so far as it is permissible to extend the definition of anxiety given in the preceding paragraph to include cases which lack one of its chief characteristics, psycho-motor excitation.

H

The sixth and last complex type of the first rank is active but unproductive mania which also occurs fairly often. Here, intellectual vacancy and verbo - motor excitation are present at the same time and are seen in inarticulate cries, singing, whistling and cheering.

The two last complex types described above have also well-known physiological counterparts in normal moods. Certainly we all know inner anxiety by experience. And we can recognize noisy unproductive joy in our daily intercourse with people who have not been forced by their upbringing or by their own common-sense to modify this complex mood which may at times become rather troublesome to those around them. We find quite a number of people whose good humour is made known by whistling, humming and restless noisy movements.

It is especially true of those forms of mood-psychosis (manic as well as melancholic) which have intellectual productivity as an integral component, that, as every mental specialist will have noticed, usually they have a certain monotony ; often the patient's range of ideas is very limited, and he will always return to it at once if he has for a moment been enticed away by his volatility of thought. The productivity, the increase of intellectual activity is as it were partial, and limited to a comparatively small circle of ideas.

We often see a completely similar phenomenon in physiological conditions, and it is this limited intellectual content of the mood that causes by its variety the many nuances found both in depressive and manic conditions, in unhappy and in cheerful moods alike. If the thoughts of a melancholy person are chiefly occupied with the past, with a loss which he has suffered, or with a fault which he has committed, his feelings will assume the character of grief, shame or despair ; if his depressive thoughts are concerned chiefly with the present and future, his feelings will be called worry, fear, anxiety or terror. In the same way states of pleasure have different characteristics partly according to whether the content of their intellectual element is something past, present or future, for example, satisfaction over something past, happiness in the present, or joyful anticipation.

Just as intellectual productivity is often limited to a small region, motor excitation, if this is part of the condition, may be limited to one or another special psycho-motor area. For example we may see an anxious or despairing patient sitting or lying in bed without the smallest tendency to change his position or to get out of bed, while the expression of his motor-excitation is limited to ceaseless hasty wringing of the hands, scratching his head, sucking his lips or constant rubbing or

59

pulling at the arm of a chair or the corner of the bed. At the same time he may even be so inhibited in the remaining motor region that he cannot be made to move from one place. We may find a corresponding motor over-activity, also only partial, in active maniacs. The varying extent of motor excitation in different cases also causes by its differing localization the great variations which may be found in states of feeling.

It would therefore be possible to develop and supplement the analysis given here of the various simple depressive and exalted states and the demonstration of the corresponding physiological feelings and moods ; anyone can, however, undertake such an elaboration, and therefore we shall not go further into the matter here. I shall only add that quite possibly someone may object to the names given by me to the different states of feeling ; it is always possible to quarrel about the meaning of the various terms and about the dividing line between the different types. Possibly there is a great difference between the meanings given by different people to words like anxiety, despair, shame, remorse, or to hope and contentment, more especially as there are of course stages of transition between them and combinations of them, and the matter is made more difficult by the inaccuracy of ordinary speech. But even if I do not always secure agreement about the nomenclature of the contents of the various categories within the scheme outlined above, that of course does not decrease the theoretical importance of these groups. They are absolutely essential to demonstrate my theory.

The six manic-melancholic intermediate types described above have been classed by me as complex types of the first order because their feeling-element is undivided whether it is exalted or depressed and has therefore a unity of feeling-tone; and similarly all normal feelings and moods corresponding to these may be called states of feeling of the first order.

Leaving these we now proceed to consider the more complicated normal and abnormal moods of the second order, *i.e.* those in which the element of feeling has two tones and shows pleasure and displeasure simultaneously.

The most typical and at the same time the most instructive manic-depressive type of the second order is pathological anger. Anger is a very comprehensive word and idea; it is used of states which may differ very widely in their inward and outward manifestation and therefore, of course, also in the physiological factors by which they are conditioned. Under the idea anger feelings are included (to take extreme examples) which may appear as rage and fury characterized by self-feeling, verbosity and aggressive tendencies, or which may be expressed in taciturn and rigidly quiet bitterness and harshness.

On this account Carl Lange is right to some extent and in respect of certain types, when he places anger next to joy in his system, because they resemble one another in outward appearance ; but the mental specialist was equally right who once declared to me that anger in his opinion has a preponderatingly depressive character and should therefore be regarded as an emotion considerably nearer to grief. The reason for this is simply that between the two extreme forms of anger there lies a whole gamut of moods differing very little one from the other, and that anger is a collective expression for a group of feelings and moods, all of which are characterized by the combination, or rather the simultaneous presence, of pleasure and unpleasure conflicting with one another in varying degrees. A mental specialist has daily opportunity of observing how close the expansive type of anger is to joy ; every day we often see our maniac patients pass for very little cause from an exalted mood to anger and back again ; and an experienced psychological investigator can hardly be in doubt as to what is happening here : into the previously unmixed feeling of pleasure there comes a more or less dominating tone of unpleasure, called forth by and directed against anyone or anything who arouses the patient's discomfort and displeasure (unpleasure).

This angry mania is therefore exactly like active productive mania with this difference, that in the former a more or less prevailing alteration has taken place in one part of the feeling-element ; the mood is no longer entirely pleasure. This expansive anger, this emotion which is chiefly pleasure with a more or less strongly marked addition of displeasure, is so usual in mania that it really belongs to the standard type of mania ; and it appears not only as a more or less transitory phase of mania but frequently as its only form during the whole course of the disease. Therefore, although it is essentially different from true mania, psychiatry has no special name for it but classes it with mania. There is, however no objection to this, as long as we are clear that there really is a difference between the two and know wherein that difference lies.

Besides this expansive anger there may also be found among disorders of mood, sometimes as a short phase and sometimes as the only form of the disease, states of mania with a more or less preponderating addition of displeasure. I refer among others to those types of pathological anger which are more like grief—types which correspond to that form of anger mentioned by my colleague quoted above. The more strongly the factor

63

of displeasure in anger is emphasized, the more it assumes the character of annoyance, bad humour, bitterness, irritation, readiness to take offence, or obstinacy, *i.e.* it approaches nearer and nearer to real anger and coincides with it as soon as the last tone of pleasure-feeling has disappeared.

In all these nuances of anger, the depressive part of the feeling-elements occupies itself of course with the thought of the cause or the object of anger, while the factor of pleasure is concerned with the idea of the angry man himself and his position as the person who is in the right and who therefore (at any rate morally speaking) can think of himself as the superior party, perhaps punishing and chastising.

Every mental specialist has come across cases of mood-psychosis in which he has hesitated whether to diagnose mania or melancholia. The displeasure-feeling has perhaps been very prominent, but the bad-humoured, peevish, argumentative, self-opinionated patient with his delight in contradiction and criticism and his inclination to annoy, irritate and plague those around him, has yet given evidence at the same time of so many factors reminiscent of mania that the doctor's uncertainty was quite explicable and justifiable.

We see from this that within the limits of the typical manic-depressive complex form of the second order, *i.e.* pathological anger, there

64

is to be found a gradual gentle transition from
the expansive forms bordering on true mania
through those which are gloomier and combined with increasing displeasure to those
depressive states which are more like true
melancholia. The most prominent and characteristic difference between them lies therefore
in the different manner in which their simultaneous pleasure and displeasure conflict with
one another ; but also the varying behaviour
of both motor and intellectual elements
provides the condition for such a number of
variations that speech can hardly find a name
for each. In the forms of pathological anger
closest to mania we shall probably most often
find motor over-activity and more or less
strongly marked flight of ideas, while in the
majority of the more depressive forms we
shall more probably find motor and intellectual
passivity or even inhibition ; but otherwise
every conceivable variation is possible.

All that we have said above of the group of
complex types of the second order of disorders
of mood, which are summed up as pathological
anger, is true, in a lesser degree, of the corresponding normal complex moods of the second
order, in so far as they are allowed to develop
unhindered by outside considerations and
circumstances, which does not often happen.
If by analysis of these moods and feelings as
they develop pathologically without regard to
anything else, we have learned to know their

constitution, we shall be able to recognize them easily in the corresponding normal states of feeling where details are less obvious and at times are distorted by considerations which do not really concern them. This group of moods under the heading anger, which extends over a wide field to rage on the one side and bad humour on the other, and borders at these extremes on the two completed pleasure- and displeasure-states, *i.e.* joy and grief, is a typical and specially instructive group of complex feelings of the second order.

Besides anger, we know a set of other feelings and moods which in their usually complex form may also be included in the same order because they are characterized by the simultaneous presence of pleasure and displeasure conflicting in various degrees. I refer to states of feeling such as longing, pensive sadness, resignation, sympathy, compassion, envy, gratitude, hope, disappointment, etc. In the analysis of all these we find at the same time pleasure and displeasure ; in some pleasure preponderates, and in others displeasure ; and in these states of feeling with a preponderance of one tone and a small addition of its opposite it seems as if this very addition of the opposite mood gives by contrast a relief and a depth to the principal feeling-tone which are lacking in states of feeling of one tone only. For example, hope is as a rule principally a feeling

66

of pleasure connected with the thought of some good which is desired and expected, but in it there is a more or less obvious displeasure-tone called forth by the thought that the hope may be disappointed. Were this dis-pleasure-tone absent, we should not be able to call the feeling hope ; it would also not have the depth and richness which makes hope superior to an unmixed pleasure-feeling. Dis-appointment is chiefly a displeasure-feeling of which the intensity depends partly on the more or less definite pleasure-tone which it also contains and which is connected with the thought of what was hoped for but not obtained.

With reference to all these terms it must be made clear that they, like anger, are really collective terms for groups of states which may indeed be closely connected and resemble one another, but may also differ very consider-ably. For example, gratitude, as a rule, is probably principally a feeling of pleasure in which the pleasure is connected with the thought of the person who has been helpful in a difficult situation and the thought that this situation is successfully over ; but in addition a displeasure-tone will be more or less clearly felt at the thought that one was not able to cope with the situation oneself and so has become as it were indebted to and dependent on someone else. In certain forms of gratitude this displeasure may be very obvious and may actually dominate the pleasure-feeling to such an extent that this gratitude may appear as a feeling chiefly of displeasure, and when the pleasure-tone finally disappears, every characteristic of gratitude is lost and the feeling coincides with grief over one's powerlessness and dependence.

A more thorough analysis will, however, reveal the fact that many of these states of feeling which are apparently complex types of the second order, are really complex types of the third, fourth or even higher orders, because their feeling-element proves to be divided not into two, but into three, four, or more simultaneous feeling-tones, and each of these tones is connected with its own part of the frequently many-sided intellectual content of the state of feeling. In a feeling such as longing we may first notice a strong pleasure-tone at the idea of the object of longing, and then a possibly very strong displeasure at the idea of having to do without it ; at the same time perhaps a more or less obvious feeling of pleasure at the thought of a possible approaching meeting and a slight displeasure at the idea that the meeting may last only a short time, and in addition perhaps a certain displeasure, connected with the memory of a slight disagreement between oneself and the object of longing at the last meeting, which by contrast increases the feeling of pleasure that the parting was very friendly, and so on.

If we investigate more closely feelings such as those above which apparently belong to the second order (and in a few cases may be proved really to belong there) it will be found that they actually belong as a rule to a much higher order because much more than two different grades of feeling occur simultaneously or in quick succession and make them more strongly differentiated and more richly faceted. The more the intellectual side of mental life is developed and cultured, the more simultaneous and different shades of feeling will a man's moods be able to include. In extremely reflective natures the strong differentiation of the feeling-element may occur at the expense of the principal feeling-tone and the result may be that the latter will be less satisfied and may be mixed with other comparatively numerous feeling-tones ; in this case the principal feeling may appear (and really be) less complete and sincere than in less complex intellects.

Among states of feeling there is a group which has a special position of its own, but is close to the feelings in its intensity and duration. We call this group the passions. It is not easy to give an exact definition of what we understand by passions or to point out exactly where they may be included among the states of feeling ; but that is as a matter of fact unnecessary.

EMOTION AND INSANITY

If we apply to the passions the same systematic principle of classification as to the feelings, love will take a place corresponding to that given above to the satisfied pleasure-feeling, joy ; and abhorrence will be the diametrical opposite of love just as the satisfied displeasure-feeling, grief, is of joy. Love and abhorrence may therefore be classified as passions of the first order.

As a passion of the second order taking a place in the classification corresponding to that of anger among the feelings, we find hatred, which is characterized by having at the same time pleasure and displeasure conflicting with one another. Analogous to anger, hatred therefore is a collective term for a number of complex passions of the second degree, which border in one direction on love, in the other on abhorrence.

As I pointed out above, in my analysis of mood-psychoses as well as of the corresponding physiological states of feeling, I have been obliged to have recourse to a simplification and schematization which is not found in real life, in order to make my views as clear as possible. It is quite obvious that in real life it is hardly ever possible to find such simple and uncomplicated states as those which have been described above as moods, feelings and emotions of the first or second order—except perhaps in the case of children

70

or of very naïve, primitive and uncivilized people. Among intellectually developed adult individuals these states, which for the sake of classification have been in the first and second order, usually prove on closer examination to be much more complex and of a much higher order.

In grief, which was mentioned above as the prototype of a satisfied displeasure-feeling of the first order (for example, the grief at the loss of a dear relative), there is in reality besides the main displeasure-tone connected with the thought of the loss, a considerable pleasure in the memory of the deceased as an expression of one's love for him ; and the stronger this pleasure-feeling is, the more sharply will it cause the displeasure-feeling at the loss to stand out as it were in relief ; but in these two dominating feeling-tones there may be further a certain pleasure-tone at the thought that the deceased is freed from his suffering and perhaps also at the idea that by his death one is oneself freed from various burdens and obligations, and further, a certain displeasure at the thought that a happy and harmonious home has been broken up by this calamity, as well as a pleasure-tone at the thought that one's own circumstances may perhaps be improved by a legacy, and to this may be added some displeasure at the thought of duties and burdens of other kinds which will devolve on one in consequence of this death, and so on.

EMOTION AND INSANITY

A passion such as love is also in very few cases of the first order—pure pleasure. As a rule many differing tones of pleasure and displeasure may play a part in it. In the first place there is a pleasure-feeling at the idea of the beloved object and possibly also at the thought of being beloved oneself ; doubt and uncertainty may however introduce a very strong displeasure-tone, and stronger or weaker displeasure-tones may be roused by jealousy, worry about the health of the beloved, opposition from others, and similar causes. And it is true of love as of feelings on the whole that the feeling-tones which contrast with the principal feeling, cause to a great extent its duration and intensity. It is a well-known fact that the more love is pleasurably satisfied, *i.e.* happy, the sooner it dies away and becomes flat, dull, insipid and empty, while in unhappy love the pleasure-feeling seems to become stronger and more intense, it lasts longer and is continually stimulated by the displeasure-tone mingled with it.

At the beginning of this chapter I emphasized the necessity of making use of certain abstract methods in our investigation, inasmuch as we should be obliged to treat and analyse as states (*i.e.* stable and unchanging) phenomena which in reality are processes (*i.e.* continually changing and advancing), but in any case I have made this obvious in my

72

analyses. The feeling-states are therefore in reality feeling-processes. And when I speak, as I did above, of grief at the loss of a dear relative, it is not a case of something stable and unchanging, but of a process occurring over a space of time and in continual change, in which pleasure- and displeasure-tones, the dominating elements in feeling-processes, change, succeed one another and coincide according to the intellectual element or elements which are each moment in the forefront of consciousness ; yet in such a way that the gradually fading feeling-tones of past processes may still make themselves felt after their intellectual content has receded in consciousness behind others. For example, in grief the chief displeasure-tone connected with the loss of the deceased, will still be felt and will to some extent affect the content of consciousness, without the memory of the death being necessarily always present. We know that this is true also of many other feelings and moods.

With regard to the relationship between the many different feeling-tones which may occur in the same feeling-process, certain psychological writers have tried to distinguish between different types in which the simultaneous feeling-tones are more or less thoroughly mixed or blended. We must, however, remember that in employing words like mixture and blending for psychical phenomena we are using metaphors taken from the material world which do not explain in the least what really happens in the psychic phenomena to which they are applied. Words like mixture and blending are in any case rather ambiguous ; we speak of mixtures of gases and liquids, but also of mixtures of powdery substances and various larger objects such as grain and fruits ; and also of mixtures of groups of people, races, etc. ; and it would be useless to argue as to which type of mixture most resembles the relationship between the simultaneous feeling-tones in a mood. The same is also more or less true of the word blending.

The most important factors in the relationship between the two feeling-tones in the same mental process seem to me to be their difference in intensity, and their extent and completeness which depends on the extent of the intellectual content with which each of them is connected. But I cannot see that apart from these factors anything else can play any part in their mutual relationship except the circumstance whether they are simultaneous, or almost simultaneous (one tone beginning before the previous one has ceased), or whether they succeed one another and in that case how quickly and frequently this happens. However tempting it may be to investigate more feeling-processes from these standpoints, it would certainly take too long and would give rise to wearisome repetition. An analysis of this kind offers indeed no very great difficulties if one bears in mind the fact that feelings, moods and emotions like all other psychical phenomena are not states but processes, and that the feeling-element in them is as a rule composed of countless feeling-tones both of pleasure and displeasure, from the mutual interplay of which there arises the resultant more or less many-sided feeling.

The analysis undertaken in this chapter of the mental disorders of mood and their really countless complex types, and also the corresponding physiological moods, feelings and emotions show us that all these (however complex they may be proved and however qualitatively different they may *appear* to be) in the last resort differ only quantitatively; and that the difference between them (apart of course from the intellectual content of each) rests only on a difference of quantity in the three elementary psychic activities, thought, psycho-motor innervation and feeling. Whatever feeling-process we investigate, it will be seen that it differs from all other such processes only in increased or decreased feeling, increased or decreased motor activity, and increased or decreased intellectual activity; or (as I have expressed it elsewhere) human emotion is the expression of the quantitative side of mental life. Its differences rest exclusively on quantitative differences in the activity of the cerebral cortex, or rather, of its centres. This will cause no surprise if we regard psychical processes as the correlative of the activity of the cerebral cortex and treat this as an organ or collection of organs which is subject to the same physiological laws as all other living organs. For of these the fundamental law holds good that whatever kind of stimulus may affect them, they are, under physiological conditions, able to respond to it only by an increase or decrease of the specific function of each particular organ.

I have concerned myself in the foregoing remarks exclusively with the psychic constituents of our feeling-processes, and in order to obtain a better general view I have purposely omitted the constituents of those which appear as changes in condition of the skin or the mucous membrane, in the activity of the alimentary canal and the various glands and in the condition of the circulatory system. I by no means undervalue, however, the importance of these ' bodily ' changes as essential parts of our feelings and emotions. Carl Lange was the first to maintain the importance of these bodily changes in human emotions. He upheld this view in his *Über Gemütsbewegungen* (1885) and aroused a storm of which it may be said that its waves have not yet subsided. I have shown elsewhere that Lange in this work goes too far in that he ignores the psychic element of feeling. But even though in his final conclusions he is not and cannot be right, it will always be his chief merit that he was the first to force us to treat psychic phenomena from a physiological point of view.

If I do not enter here into a discussion of these bodily changes, it is because they are of comparatively little importance for the purpose of this work and because their inclusion in my analysis would make the latter too detailed and lacking in clearness.

As for the varying behaviour of the circulatory system in the different feeling-processes, it has been discussed in the last decades to a quite disproportionate extent and an importance has been given to it which it by no means deserves. Moreover these investigations and measurements of the changes in the circulatory organs have been too often misused by experimentalists who, in the interpretation of their extremely ambiguous graphs and tables have lacked that indispensable corrective to their experiments which comes from a thorough physiological training, and who therefore usually arrive at results which contradict all physiology.

It will have been noticed that in the analysis of the mood-psychoses and of normal feeling-processes, I have consistently grouped together the quantitative changes in the psychic elements of which, as we have found, they are composed. There is an impulse in human nature to seek a certain relationship, a causal connection between simultaneous or almost simultaneous phenomena and to assume or maintain causal connection without sufficient investigation if the theory sounds plausible. This tendency has shown itself also in the general conception of feelings, moods and emotions, and especially in the connection between their various component parts. Both in daily speech and in literature it happens extraordinarily often that in the discussion or description of a state of feeling one or more integral parts of it are singled out and considered to be the product of the state of feeling. People say that grief *acts* on thought or on power of action with paralysing effect; or that a shock *makes* one speechless; an author may say of the person whom he is describing that anxiety *drives* him up and down the room perplexed and wringing his hands, or that anger *causes* him to clench his fists or stamp on the floor, or he may say of a child or a girl that joy *makes* her shout, clap her hands, dance about, and so on. We are here assuming a causal connection of which even in the most favourable circumstances we know nothing. We imagine that we are giving an explanation whereas in reality it is incomprehensible why and how it happens that grief

78

should have a paralysing effect and anxiety quite the contrary. It is indeed no explanation to assume a causal connection between these phenomena ; none of them becomes more comprehensible by this means. Owing to the insight into the various states of feeling and their constitution, which we have gained by our previous analysis of them into their component elements, we can on the contrary maintain that, for example, the inhibition (both intellectual and psycho-motor) in grief is not a product of grief but an integral part which is connected with the depressive feeling of displeasure and is equally important for the inner and the outer manifestation of the whole feeling-state. If the motor and intellectual inhibition is taken from grief, it is no longer grief, because the latter is characterized by inhibition, but a more indefinite displeasure-feeling ; or if the flight of ideas and the motor-excitation are removed which drive the anxious man up and down wringing his hands, it will no longer be anxiety but only a certain displeasure which differs in no way from the feeling which remains when inhibition is removed from grief. We must therefore consider it unjustifiable to remove from a state of feeling one or more of its integral indispensable parts and call them its product.

Of course I do not wish to prevent daily speech or poetic language from making use of such descriptive phrases as the above. That would be as absurd and useless as to try to prevent people in general and writers in particular from speaking, for example, of the rising and setting of the sun, although we all know that it is the earth which revolves.

It is quite a different matter when it is a question of scientific investigation of feeling-states and their abnormal exaggerations, the different types of manic-depressive psychosis. In such an investigation it is of course not practicable to attribute scientific value to popular views or to phrases of daily speech. And yet in the scientific treatment of these states we find a tendency exactly similar to the popular view mentioned above. Various writers on psychiatry adopt it, and in their description and analysis of melancholy and mania they maintain that there is a causal connection between the psychic changes of mania and melancholy similar in every way to that attributed to the different normal moods by daily speech. It sounds quite plausible and suits the popular idea of the connection quite well when people say that in melancholy it is the depressive mood, displeasure, which *acts* with inhibitive force on the movements and thoughts of the melancholic; or that the exalted mood, the increased pleasure-feeling, is the *cause* of the flight of ideas and the urge to movement of the maniac. But as I have said above, the causal connection cannot be proved and its assumption is unjustifiable.

80

It should in reality be quite as justifiable to maintain (as Fr. Lange does in his " Geistes-krankheitsgruppen ") the exact opposite, *i.e.* that the intellectual and motor inhibition is the cause of the depressed mood in melancholy, and not the other way about.

Meanwhile, however, none of the various writers gives any explanation of how it happens and why a depressed mood should cause inhibition and vice versa, and a cheerful mood have the contrary effect ; they simply state it as something self-evident which every one must be able to understand. But not only is this assertion not provable, it also obviously contradicts the knowledge gained from our study of the manic-melancholic complex types. Even if there really existed in mental disorders of mood or in normal moods a causal connection between the changes in the feeling-element and the changes in the other psychic elements, we should have of necessity to prove a certain conformity to law in the connection between cause and effect according to which pleasure or displeasure would always produce the same effects in the intellectual and psycho-motor sphere ; so that, for example, displeasure would always cause inhibition and pleasure the contrary.

The study of manic-depressive complex conditions gives, however, abundant proof that such a conformity to law does not really exist, and that quite the contrary is true.

Among the countless complex types of mania-melancholia we find for example a depressed mood (displeasure) sometimes united with intellectual and motor inhibition as in passive unproductive melancholia, sometimes with motor excitation and with or without intellectual hyper-function as in anxiety-melancholia. Then again we see a cheerful mood (pleasure) sometimes united with excitement as in typical mania, sometimes with motor inhibition and with changes in one direction or the other of the intellectual functions as in passive, stupid, more or less productive mania ; in short, there is really no quantitative change in the intellectual and motor sphere which may not be found connected sometimes with pleasure, sometimes with displeasure.

It must, then, be accepted as clearly proved that change in the feeling-element, whether in positive or negative direction, cannot be the cause of changes in the intellectual or motor sphere and vice versa, and that on the contrary the changes in all three psychic elements must be co-ordinate component parts of the single state of feeling. This is of course also true of the physiological moods, feelings and emotions which correspond to the various pathological disorders of mood.

If this has been clearly understood, then, it will also be obvious that exactly the same is true of all the various ' bodily ' changes

PSYCHIATRY AND PSYCHOLOGY

which we see in the different states of feeling. According to the popular view and the usual way of speaking, we are inclined to attribute to these also a causal connection with the psychic elements in the states of feeling. In melancholia and grief we usually find a decrease in the function of the alimentary canal which appears as constipation and loss of appetite, and at the same time there is often decreased secretion in the sweat- and saliva-glands ; in states of mania and of joy we often find great activity of the intestines, increased secretion of the various glands, and so on ; in states of anxiety and other complex types there are various combinations of these bodily changes. But none of these changes is *caused* by melancholia or mania, any more than they are (as Carl Lange tried to prove) causes of the feeling-states. On the contrary all of them are integral and equally important parts of the mood or disease, like the changes in the feeling-element, in thought and in mobility. The same is also true, of course, of all the changes in the blood-pressure, in respiration and in the condition of the pulse, which may be tested by the help of various measuring apparatus. These are also characteristic and are co-ordinate with the other component parts of the single feelings and moods.

Probably the chief reason why people have been tempted to ascribe a certain causal

83

connection to the different changes which constitute a state of feeling, is the fact that they do not appear simultaneously. It must, however, be remembered, as I have emphasized above, that all these feelings and moods are not states which are finished and rounded off, but that here we are dealing with processes which are progressing and passing ; of course there is nothing to prevent one part of these from appearing earlier or later than another, but it should not therefore be assumed that the part which appears first is the cause of the later one.

Just as, for example, displeasure in melancholia, grief or anxiety is not the cause of the quantitative changes in psycho-motility and thought contained in these states, so also displeasure or these changes are not the causes of all the ' bodily ' changes belonging to melancholia, grief or anxiety ; all these effects (those of the feeling-element as well as those of the circulatory system and the glands) are of equal rank even though they do not always appear simultaneously, and they are due to the same central cause, *i.e.* the impression which has called forth the mood or feeling.

To give a physiological explanation of why and how it happens that one impression should cause the set or series of quantitative organic changes which constitute joy, and another, all those which produce the type of anger, anxiety or grief, is beyond human ability and probably will always remain so. We must bow to that as to any other fact. It simply is so. But in any case we get no nearer to an understanding of it if we assume a causal connection between the various component parts, a connection which cannot be proved, which explains nothing but contradicts the knowledge gained by psychiatry through the study of the complex types of manic-depressive psychosis, and which, as we have seen by means of the light cast on the physiological life of feeling by this study, holds good also for normal moods, feelings and emotions.

PHYSIOLOGY

CHAPTER IV

As we have seen in the preceding chapters, the fundamental idea in the present work is that moods, feelings and emotions correspond, as regards their psychic constituents, to cerebral activity, or, more exactly, to the functioning of cells in the grey matter of the cerebrum, and that the cerebral cortex as a bodily organ must follow the physiological laws which govern all living organs.

We have now reached that point in the development of our theme at which we must proceed to apply these physiological laws to the knowledge gained through our investigation of human feelings from the standpoint of psychiatry and psychology.

One general law which holds good in the whole human body is that specifically different functions are always fulfilled by specifically different cells ; contraction of the muscles is always caused by muscle-cells, saliva is produced by the salivary gland-cells, urine by the cells of the kidneys, and so on. We must therefore logically conclude that specifically different cerebral functions must be exercised by specifically different brain-cells.

In confirmation of this, modern microscopic examination of the brain has succeeded in showing decided differences in the structure of the different regions of the cerebral cortex (cf. Brodmann), and it is not at all unreasonable to look upon these anatomical differences as the expression of corresponding physiological differences, *i.e.* differences in function. The brain is really to be regarded as a complexity of organs, each of which has its special function, while their close anatomical connection is the expression of their close physiological association.

In the chapter on Psychology we succeeded in proving—and in the chapter on Psychiatry and Psychology we confirmed the fact—that in every mental product three specifically distinct elementary psychic functions are found. And in accordance with the fundamental law mentioned above we must conclude that each of these is fulfilled by its particular type of cells, which are grouped each within its special organ within the organ-complex of the cerebral cortex. It is many years since the position of the organ of psycho-motor innervation was determined. It is situated in the ascending frontal convolution and in the course of time it has been possible to differentiate in detail between the motor centres of the various parts of the body.

PHYSIOLOGY

As far as the intellectual functions are concerned, we know with certainty some of the positions of the sense-centres. The centre of sight lies in the occipital lobes ; the centre of hearing in the temporal region ; the tactile centres of the different parts of the skin are to be found in the parietal convolution near the corresponding motor-centres of those parts in the frontal convolution ; and the centres of the sense of pain are probably close to the centres of touch.

With regard to the higher intellectual functions or thought proper, there are various reasons for believing that this takes place in the frontal region of the brain, or, to be more exact, in the two upper frontal convolutions, the third being chiefly concerned with the speech-centre (Broca's centre). Opinion is still divided, however, as to whether the frontal region is the seat of the intellect.

Only the position of the centre of elementary feeling is completely uncertain. But that feeling, as an elementary psychic activity, must correspond to the function of particular brain-cells collected in one centre, seems to me self-evident after the preceding explanation ; any other assumption would be quite unphysiological and would contradict especially the main physiological law quoted above which holds good for all human organs, i.e. the law of the specific energy of the living cell.

We shall, however, at this point discuss the

assumption that feeling has not a centre of its own but is a by-product of cells with a different main function, *i.e.* intellectual activity (sensation or idea), as this theory has been advanced by certain psycho-physiologists.

In a treatise published in 1892 on the Laws of Human Feeling * Alfred Lehmann, rejecting the theory of a special centre of feeling, put forward the following hypothesis concerning the origin of the psychic element of feeling, that " pleasure is the psychic consequence of the fact that an organ while working does not use up a greater amount of energy than nutrition can replace ; displeasure on the other hand is the psychic consequence of every disproportion between consumption and nutrition, as it arises both when the consumption of energy exceeds the supply and when the supply, by reason of the inactivity of the organ, exceeds the maximum which can be received."

In my treatise on the Manic-depressive Psychosis (1902) already referred to, I tried to show that this theory is untenable. I maintained that pleasure cannot be the psychic consequence of an equilibrium of consumption and nutrition, and in proving this I pointed to the fact that every one experiences a greater or a lesser feeling of pleasure while we cannot imagine a greater or lesser equilibrium ; pleasure cannot therefore be an

* *Die Hauptgesetze des menschlichen Gefühlslebens.*

expression for equilibrium. And displeasure
cannot correspond to a lack of equilibrium in
one direction or the other between consumption and nutrition, for then we should certainly be able to feel two kinds of displeasure,
one aroused by the excess of consumption
over supply, and the other by the opposite.
But we know only one kind of displeasure-
feeling. Moreover, in any case the first type
of displeasure could only be of quite short
duration, while life often shows us extremely
tedious displeasure-states ; and it is impossible
to understand how the other kind of displeasure-feeling could arise.

About the same time, however, or, to be
more exact, shortly before this, Lehmann
somewhat modified his view and formulated
his dynamic theory of feeling thus : " When
a psycho-physiological process demands from
each functioning neurone no greater expenditure of energy than can be replaced continually
by metabolism, its psychic effect will be a
pleasure-feeling while its physiological effect
will be to open the way for movements in
other centres. The highest feeling of pleasure
will be obtained when it is possible for metabolism exactly to cover the expenditure of
energy. If this limit is passed, both the
pleasure-feeling and the possibility of movement in other centres will quickly decrease,
because the expenditure in the functioning
centre calls forth a flow of energy from its

environment, and therefore in the latter simultaneous processes are inhibited. Under these conditions the psychic state is at first neutral, tending sometimes towards pleasure, sometimes towards displeasure, according to circumstances. If finally the expenditure in the functioning neurones becomes so great that it cannot be made good by metabolism in conjunction with the intercellular flow of energy, the psychic effect will then be a displeasure-feeling." *

If from all these circumlocutions we extract the main idea, we have the following result : pleasure arises when metabolism in the brain is able continuously to replace the consumption of the brain-cells, and the highest pleasure-feeling is reached when metabolism is able to cover the exact loss. I must confess that I am incapable of seeing any difference between replacing and covering in this connection ; according to common usage the meaning is the same, *i.e.* that supply and consumption balance one another ; pleasure would therefore always be identical with the highest pleasure. This theory allows only one degree of pleasure, the maximum, whereas anyone with any power of introspection knows different degrees of pleasure. In reality, therefore, the explanation of the dynamic theory of feeling proves, as regards pleasure, to be the

* *Die körperlichen Äusserungen psychischer Zustände*, Part II, Leipzig, 1901.

94

same as in the theory of 1892 and is to be met by the same objection : pleasure cannot correspond to such an equilibrium for this cannot increase or diminish as pleasure can according to universal experience.

In this later formulation of the theory, displeasure is no longer said to have two sources, but arises only from the inability of metabolism together with an intercellular flow of energy to make good the consumption of the cell. It does not seem to me that the theory is improved by the introduction of an intercellular flow of energy ; even in this form it permits displeasure to be a process of only quite short duration, whereas in life both outside and inside asylums we know of such lasting and obstinate displeasure-states that we cannot possibly imagine them to arise from a continual deficiency of supply to the functioning brain-cells. It cannot, therefore, be maintained that Lehmann has been more fortunate in his obscurely formulated dynamic theory of 1901 than in the original hypothesis of 1892.

Nevertheless, in his later publications * on this subject he maintains his dynamic theory of feeling with only very slight improvements (but with omission of the intercellular flow of energy) and supports it according to Berger's

---

* *Elemente der Psychodynamik*, 1905 ; *Grundzüge der Psychophysiologie*, 1912 ; and the second edition of *Die Hauptgesetze des menschlichen Gefühlslebens*, 1914.

method by Verworn's mistaken (as we shall see later) study of Biotonus. In its latest formulation (1914) the dynamic theory of feeling runs thus : " When during the activity of a central group of neurones the assimilation is equal to the dissimilation, $\frac{A}{D}=I$, this condition makes itself felt psychically as pleasure, which increases according to the increase of value of the dissimilation and assimilation. If, however, the dissimilation is greater than the assimilation, and the biotonus therefore decreases, $\frac{A}{D}<I$, this condition is realized psychically as displeasure which increases according as the value of $\frac{A}{D}$ decreases." We see here that Lehmann persists in thinking that the physiological basis of pleasure is that the supply (assimilation) of the nerve-cells is equal to their consumption (dissimilation), *i.e.* that these are equally balanced. But at the same time we see that, in order to avoid the difficulty that an equilibrium cannot increase and decrease, he makes a sudden evasion by stating that the pleasure-feeling increases and decreases, not according to the equilibrium of which he alleges it is the psychic expression but according to something quite different, the compensatory function of the cells themselves. This position is however quite untenable ; he must make his choice between the

two. Either the pleasure-feeling corresponds to this equilibrium and must increase and decrease with it, which is impossible ; or else pleasure increases and decreases with the rise or fall in the compensated functioning of the cell ; and in that case pleasure is a direct product of the cell or rather a by-product, for the cell according to Lehmann has quite a different main function, *i.e.* sensation or ideation.

But even if anything so contrary to physiology were to be admitted as that the same cell should have two different elementary functions, such as feeling and intellectual activity, (a phenomenon otherwise quite unknown in the human organism), that would not help this theory in the least ; for it will be seen that it is in its first corollaries in irreconcilable conflict with the experience of everyday life. The main corollaries to be deduced from Lehmann's theory are the three following :

1. Increasing intellectual activity (*i.e.* increasing intensity of sensation and ideation) *must* always cause increase of pleasure.

2. Two sense-impressions of the same intensity must always have the same feeling-tone.

3. A sensation or idea cannot have a dis-

pleasure-tone without having just had a pleasure-tone, or indeed without having passed through a certain maximum of pleasure.

Lehmann himself realizes these logical consequences of the dynamic theory of feeling and searches eagerly for examples which may support them while he resolutely closes his eyes to all the daily facts which contradict them. In support of the first of these three corollaries of his theory Lehmann maintains that the pleasure-tone of a sensation always increases according to the intensity of the stimulus which calls forth that sensation and that this holds good for all the senses. This is a bold statement, but it is false. Strong colours *can* certainly have a stronger pleasure-tone than the corresponding weaker ones ; but the opposite is the case at least as often. Many people, and not necessarily those with the worst taste, decidedly prefer delicate colours to the corresponding strong ones, without on that account finding the latter ugly. In their case, therefore, a dynamic theory of feeling does not hold good. The same is true of sounds ; a note *may* sometimes, when it is struck loudly, have a stronger pleasure-tone than when it is struck gently ; but the contrary is the case at least as often, a fact which directly contradicts Lehmann's theory. When not merely single notes but whole compositions are in question, it becomes very obvious that the theory fails when applied to auditory sensations, for if dynamic force plays the chief and decisive part in their feeling-tone, as this theory of feeling asserts, it would seem that every composer and orchestral conductor would be best advised to use *fortissimo* continually ; but they do not. There is no doubt that a *crescendo* may cause increase of enjoyment ; but as often, if not more often, pleasure is increased by a *diminuendo* and culminates in a pleasure-feeling bordering on ecstasy with a dying and hardly audible *pianissimo*. That would be inconceivable if feeling-tone depended on dynamic force alone. Of course I know well that the feeling-tone of a single note as a rule plays a comparatively small part in the feeling aroused by a whole composition. But according to the dynamic theory of feeling it must be the essential thing, since the ideas and organic sensations aroused by the music are so vague and veiled, so shifting and lacking in intensity that it is inconceivable that by their dynamic force they could have any special influence on the collective feeling. Moreover it may be possible to eliminate their influence. For example, let the Garden scene from *Faust* be played twice by the same orchestra under the same conductor in exactly the same way, except that the first time it is played *pianissimo* as Gounod wrote it, and the second time *fortissimo ;* we should then see whether the dynamic theory of feeling really holds good. In that case it would really be very curious that most of the great erotic music of the world is composed for *piano* and *pianissimo* performance. Lehmann's theory, therefore, is inadequate for both sounds and colours.

It is no better when applied to the sensations of taste and smell. In these also the pleasure-tone *may* certainly increase with the intensity of the sensation but the contrary is very often the case. Every cookery-book emphasizes and every gourmand knows that in the preparation of food it is important to put in only a suggestion of certain spices and essences. Does this not depend on the fact that quite slight sensations of taste and smell have often a greater pleasure-tone than corresponding strong ones, although the latter need not necessarily be unpleasant ?

If from the simple sensations we proceed to apply the theory to higher intellectual activity, we should expect that increasing mental work would always produce an increase of pleasure. There can be no doubt that this *may* be the case, but it is certainly not always so. At least as often we notice that increasing intellectual work leaves us quite indifferent or even causes a certain displeasure-feeling, without our having any reason to suppose that there is any over-exertion of the brain-cells. The work may simply be boring. On the other hand it is quite often found that, in direct contradiction of the theory, a decrease of intellectual work causes increasing pleasure which often actually culminates in complete intellectual repose.

All these facts which directly contradict the first corollary of the dynamic theory of feeling and therefore refute it, are of such daily and common occurrence that the most casual observer can bear witness to their accuracy.

The second corollary of Lehmann's theory was that two sensations of the same intensity must always have the same feeling-tone. According to this it would be inconceivable that of two equally strong colours one should be considered beautiful (with a pleasure-tone) and the other ugly (with a displeasure-tone) ; and they must both be of exactly equal beauty according to the theory. It would also be inconceivable that one of two equally loud notes should have a slight pleasure-tone because it is in tune, and the other a strong displeasure-tone because it is out of tune. If feeling-tone were dependent on the dynamic force of the notes, it would be the same for both. Or take two equally strong sensations of taste and smell—for example, on the one hand a very slight smell or taste of vanilla and on the other a musty or rancid taste of corresponding strength. How can the dynamic theory help us to explain that the former will certainly give us considerable enjoyment while the latter will disgust us? According to the theory they should affect us in the same way. Or let us take an example from higher intellectual activity; it is hard to imagine that it is a greater strain for the brain-cells to think of an unsympathetic than of a sympathetic person, or of an unpleasant than of a pleasant event. But if it is not so, how can Lehmann explain the different feeling-tone of these ideas? We see therefore that the second corollary of the dynamic theory of feeling also contradicts the simplest daily experiences and proves it quite incapable of explaining them.

The third corollary, however, is the most fatal for Lehmann's theory, namely, that a sensation or idea cannot have a displeasure-tone without having just had a pleasure-tone and indeed having passed through a certain maximum of pleasure. This is the logical consequence of the fact that displeasure, according to Lehmann, always arises from the excess of the consumption (dissimilation) of the nerve-cells over their supply (assimilation). In order that this may happen, the activity of the cells must naturally have reached a certain quite considerable height; for it cannot well be assumed that the supply to a cell will fail at the outset. But how can we reconcile this with the fact that in the course of each day all of us experience with regard to all the senses a great number of sensations which are quite slight but nevertheless often have a very strong displeasure-tone ? A slight smell of gas or coal-smoke, a suggestion of sulphuretted hydrogen or free butyric acid, a slight smell of cabbage, garlic or cheese, and a thousand other quite slight sensations of smell may cause great discomfort to many people. The buzzing of a fly on the window-pane, the slight rattling of a window-fastening, a discordant hurdy-gurdy in the distance—these and similar sensations may cause displeasure from the first moment. The scarcely audible scratching of a knife on a nail makes me shrink and is almost sufficient to give me cold shudders ; a slight touch of woollen material on his teeth has a similar effect on one of my colleagues ; on others, a stroking of the hand over fibrous silken material ; examples *ad infinitum* may be found in daily life. How is it possible or conceivable that all these very slight sensations can cause a lack of equilibrium in the assimilation of the corresponding brain-cells, a consumption which exceeds the supply ?

Lehmann has himself seen the absurd and illogical side of his theory when applied to sensations which are quite weak in pleasure-tone and he especially realizes the difficulty of always, according to his theory, passing through a certain maximum of pleasure before displeasure is reached. He tries to

EMOTION AND INSANITY

explain the fact that certain sensations appear on the very threshold of consciousness with a displeasure-tone, by saying that the pleasure-maximum through which they must first have passed according to his theory before they can have a displeasure-tone, has already been reached, but accompanied by such a slight sensation that it was hardly felt. Will anyone really find this explanation satisfactory?

Owing to his conception of displeasure as the expression of a lack of balance in the metabolism of the brain-cells, Lehmann is forced to oppose the otherwise generally accepted view of pleasure and displeasure as greater and lesser degrees of the same psychic phenomenon. It is true that he recognizes feeling as a psychic element and pleasure and displeasure as opposites within it; but he definitely rejects the logical conclusion that they can therefore differ only in degree; according to his opinion they are on the contrary *qualitatively* different. But it is not easy to see how opposites within the same psychic phenomenon can be qualitatively different; psychology, like physiology, knows only quantitative differences of function within the same area.

In his three latest works on this subject, to which reference was made above, Lehmann attempts by means of a diagram to illustrate this idea of the relation between pleasure and displeasure, and also his conception of the transition from one to the other. But this diagram, far from illustrating his point of view, gives on the contrary an excellent graphic description of the very idea which he so obstinately contests, namely, that pleasure and displeasure are different in degree and that the transition from the highest pleasure to displeasure is made by passing through continually decreasing pleasure to a stage of complete indifference and thence to displeasure.

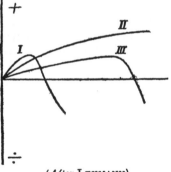

The diagram copied here is explained by Lehmann as follows : the intensity of the sensation is represented by the abscissa, the intensity of feeling as ordinate.

(*After* Lehmann)

The positive ordinates denote pleasure, the negative, displeasure.

It is obvious that this drawing and his explanation of it flatly contradict his own theory. It is impossible to illustrate two qualitatively different phenomena by placing them on the same ordinate as positive and negative respectively. Anyone who does this acknowledges by that very fact that they are qualitatively of the same nature. Moreover, according to Lehmann's diagram, whether we follow the ordinate or one of the curves representing the various sensations, it is not possible to go from the highest pleasure to the deepest displeasure without passing through a continual decrease in pleasure to a stage of indifference and thence to displeasure. According to the theory, however, one ought on the contrary to go in the opposite direction through a continual increase of pleasure reaching displeasure after passing through a maximum of pleasure. If Lehmann desired to illustrate by a diagram his own opinion of the mutual relationship of pleasure and displeasure, he should have placed the beginning of displeasure on the ordinate *above* the maximum pleasure-point. It would be difficult to find a more infelicitous diagram than Lehmann has devised in this case.

We see, therefore, that each of the corollaries to be deduced from the dynamic theory of feeling is in irreconcilable conflict with the experience of everyday life. There is therefore no reason to believe on account of its special attributes that the brain holds a special position among all living organisms, in that two essentially different elementary psychic functions such as feeling and intellectual activity are united in the same brain-cells.

In Chapter XII of his *Die Hauptgesetze des menschlichen Gefühlslebens* (1914) Lehmann mentions that some psychiatrists (Thalbitzer and Niessl-Mayendorf) assume that there is a special feeling-centre. But, he adds, we do not need to accept this, as the hypothesis was formulated in order to explain certain pathological circumstances, and a hypothesis of this kind must primarily apply to normal mental phenomena which we know far better than pathological ones ; concerning the latter we can only base assumptions on the often very scanty data collected from patients. This reasoning makes it very clear that Lehmann knows nothing of mental cases nor of the working methods of mental specialists, and that he therefore has no idea of the value of our observations for the critical examination of the normal life of feeling. At the same time his remarks betray a tendency not uncommon among psychologists, to deny the claim of mental specialists to have a voice in psychological questions.

In the same passage, Lehmann refers to my view expressed in my earlier works, that pleasure and displeasure, being opposites different only in degree within elementary feeling, must of necessity correspond to a functioning of the brain-cells which differs also only in degree. To this he raises the following objections : " Pleasure and displeasure are qualitatively different phenomena

of consciousness " ; and " Displeasure is not a
lesser degree of pleasure, any more than green
is a paler red. A theory of colours, which
tried to explain complementary colours as
degrees, differing in intensity, of the same
phenomenon, would certainly not be taken
seriously. What is true in the one case,
holds good also in the other." At the first
glance Lehmann's argument may perhaps
seem plausible, but on closer examination we
see that—whether consciously or unconsciously—it does but cleverly beg the question.
Every one must agree that pleasure and displeasure are *psychic* opposites ; even Lehmann
proceeds from this assumption, and in any
case this is presupposed by the very terms
pleasure and displeasure. But the sensation
red and the sensation green are by no means
psychic opposites. *Psychically* there is no
other or greater contrast between the sensation red and the sensation green than, for
example, between the sensations red and blue
or yellow and green ; they are merely different
colour-sensations. It would never occur to
anyone to call the sensation green a weaker
sensation of red or vice versa, or to call red
dis-green (by analogy with pleasure and displeasure) ; and therefore the sensation red
and the sensation green cannot be different
degrees of intensity of the same psychic
phenomena and so correspond to a higher
and lower function of the same brain-cells.

The relation between two complementary colours is analogous, for example, to the relation between acids and alkalis ; and there can hardly be anyone who would describe an acid taste as a weak alkali taste or vice versa. The fact that two external phenomena neutralize one another—I might almost say accidentally—chemically or in the spectrum, is of course quite irrelevant to the psychic connection between the sensations aroused by them. If we knew nothing of spectral analysis, it would never occur to us that there is a special antithetical relationship between green and red rays of light. There can therefore be no justification for the attempt to draw a parallel between pleasure-displeasure-feeling and red-green-sensation.

Lehmann then continues : " When Thal-bitzer goes on to explain pleasure as stimulation of the feeling-centre which exceeds the norm, and displeasure as one which does not reach the norm, his hypothesis becomes really unpsychological. He does not take into account even the well-known fact that displeasure as a rule accompanies the stronger stimulation." I have quoted this passage because it is a characteristic example of Lehmann's unscrupulousness in misinterpreting psychological facts when it is a question of making them fit his purpose. Here for his contention he needs the statement that " displeasure as a rule accompanies the stronger stimulation," and so he exalts that into a "well-known fact"; while even the most casual observer of life knows (and indeed it has also been amply proved in the psychological analyses of the previous chapter) that displeasure at least as often is found in conjunction with inhibition while " stimulation " is perhaps most frequently found in exalted conditions which have therefore a pleasure-tone.

Although, therefore, strictly speaking it might be considered superfluous, yet perhaps in some ways it may be interesting to examine more closely the reasons which caused Lehmann to reject from the start and so decidedly the hypothesis of a special feeling-centre. These appear with slight variations in all his works on the subject since 1892, and are found finally in Chapter XII of the second edition of the *Hauptgesetze* (1914). There are three circumstances which in his opinion contradict the theory of an independent feeling-centre ; but their insignificance is really astonishing.

The first of these is based on the phenomenon which Lehmann claims to have observed, that feeling-tone appears in consciousness at the same moment as the sensation to which it belongs. This is a mere postulate, and in view of several circumstances I am much inclined to doubt its correctness.

But even if we assume that he is right in saying that it is impossible for introspection to detect an interval between sensation and its feeling-tone, I do not see why this is an argument against an anatomically separate genesis of the two phenomena ; for even if the centres of the two psychic activities, sensation and feeling, were to be imagined as situated in opposite poles of the brain, the distance between them could not be greater than 25 cmm. ; and when we think of the great velocity of the transmission of nervous impulse (according to Tigerstedt, a velocity of between 32 and 120 metres a second), it is not surprising that so small a space of time as would here be in question, should be impossible to observe. The first reason for disputing the existence of a feeling-centre is therefore quite invalid.

Secondly, Lehmann says, all feelings and ideas may appear with a feeling-tone. Therefore nerve tracts must run from all sense-centres into this hypothetical feeling-centre ; but, he declares, "there is no such point in the cerebral cortex." That this feeling-centre must be a point is Lehmann's own invention ; it is, and always has been, my definite opinion that the feeling-centre like all other cortical centres occupies a not inconsiderable anatomical space and is composed of a sufficient number of brain-cells to fulfil this comprehensive function. And in the millions of nerve-fibres of the centrum semiovales there must certainly be enough tracts to unite such a centre with all the various sense-centres.

The last argument against the existence of a feeling-centre is as unimportant as the first two. If there were a special feeling-centre, a greater or lesser injury to that centre would cause a total or partial 'lack of feeling,' *i.e.* a lack of feeling-tone in sensations and ideas ; and that Lehmann considers to be quite inconceivable. If he had not such a great contempt for psychiatry and especially for its power of throwing light on psychological problems, he would be able to learn from any modern mental specialist that the improved clinical methods in the psychiatry of the last decades have shown that certain stationary defective conditions arising from those abnormal processes which we group under the heading dementia præcox, are especially characterized by a more or less definite dulling, decreasing or even complete loss of the emotional side of the patient's mental life. This emotional dementia is especially noticeable in those not infrequent cases in which it appears conjointly with a comparatively unimpaired intellect. And in these very cases the thought occurs to one insistently that this comparatively one-sided and specially emotional dullness must be caused by the fact that here the disease must have attacked chiefly the feeling-centre.

We must therefore consider it as definitely settled that feeling is not a by-product of brain-cells which have another function, but that if we recognize feeling to be an elementary psychic function, we must also acknowledge that it proceeds from its own cells which are collected in a feeling-centre. From the physiological point of view this centre must behave in exactly the same way as all other bodily organisms, especially in that its specific function can only increase or decrease, and this makes itself known psychically as exalted feeling (pleasure) or depressed feeling (displeasure). So far we know nothing certain of the position of this feeling-centre except that it cannot at any rate lie in an area already occupied by another function. It cannot, therefore, be found in the frontal region, which presumably contains the centres of higher intellectual activity and the speech-centre (in the third left frontal). Nor can it be in the ascending frontal convolution which is the seat of psycho-motor innervation, while the sensitive tracts of touch and probably also of pain and temperature end in the ascending parietal convolution. In the folds of the temporal lobe are situated the hearing-centres. There remains only the hinder part of the brain.

As I have indicated elsewhere, various circumstances point to the occipital lobes of the brain (Gyri occipitales) as the feeling-centre, in so far as these are not occupied by the sight-centre which is to be found on their median surface. I have also shown before that there is an anatomical fact which supports this localization, *i.e.* that the brain is provided with blood by three pairs of main arteries coming from the circle of Willis which surrounds the base of the brain, and that the front pair of these arteries carries blood to the frontal region, and the middle one to the central region and to many of the parietal and temporal convolutions, while the occipital lobes are provided with blood by the posterior pair of these great cerebral arteries. In the rest of the human body we know that the various organs are mutually independent in respect of their blood-supply, and it is probable that this holds good also in the brain and that, in other words, the region supplied by each of these pairs of arteries corresponds to the position of the centre for a particular elementary mental activity.

This demand for a localization of psychic elements might be called a kind of phrenology. And it can hardly be doubted that the fundamental idea on which the phrenology of the past was based, was quite correct. The theory of different positions for different psychic phenomena is really only an application to the brain of a fact which has been found to apply everywhere else in the human organism, *i.e.* that essentially different activities and products proceed from different and differently situated organs. The errors of phrenology come from the fact that Gall, the founder of the science, and his followers regarded single concrete psychic products as being essentially different, and they therefore thought it necessary to localize each of them. Gall, was, however, more important as a brain-anatomist than as a psychologist, and he can hardly be blamed for this, considering the condition of psychological science at that time. He and other phrenologists did not see that each of the concrete psychic products to which they allotted a position could be resolved into three essentially different psychic elements to be found in all of them ; and that there could be a question only of localizing these three elementary activities. The demand for their localization, a very reasonable one according to the arguments developed above, may then be looked upon as a sublimated phrenology, a phrenology in nobler form, which may in all respects be reconciled with the conclusions of the analytical method in empirical psychology concerning the elementary mental activities.* It was in reality a renaissance of phrenology that was introduced when Fritsch and Hitzig demonstrated the position of the psycho-motor centres in the brain.

* " We are thus once more led to assume that there is a localization, a division of work within the cerebrum, but such that only the elementary mental activities, the powers of sensation and movement, are localized " (Höffding, *Psychologie*).

The next universal physiological law which we shall discuss in its application to the brain, is the law of the ' tonus ' of living organs, a law to which enough attention is seldom paid and which is almost ignored by psycho-physiology.

Here we must first examine more closely the notion of Tonus. Literally, in its derivation from the Greek τείνειν (to stretch) the term means ' tension.' In physiology it was first used of the unstriped muscles of the vessels ; when these muscles were said to have tonus, the meaning was that as long as they are living they are always contracted to some extent. Gradually it was realized that this was true not only of vascular muscles or unstriped muscles in general, but of all transversely-striated muscles. And in the course of time it became clear not only that tonus is characteristic of muscle-cells, but that all cells as long as they are living, are functioning to some extent and have a certain tonus. Living cells never stand still but always show a certain degree of their specific function ; that is true of muscle-cells as well as of the cells belonging to the liver, the saliva glands and the kidneys, and it is of course also true of nerve-cells and brain-cells. Thus the term and the theory of tonus have by analogy been extended in a way which has been commonly accepted by scientists, and it now denotes the degree of function in which a single organ or cell is found at any moment.

PHYSIOLOGY

The well-known German physiologist, Verworn of Bonn, in his *Allgemeine Physiologie* uses and understands the word tonus differently in the development of his ' biotonus ' theory. In the life process of cells two phases can be distinguished : assimilation and dissimilation. By assimilation we mean that activity by which the cell takes from the blood and uses the materials which it needs for its special purpose ; by dissimilation we mean that activity, by which the cell changes its content into the final product characteristic of it, whether it be saliva, gall, muscular contraction or nervous impulse ; and the connection between assimilation and dissimilation (A/D) is called by Verworn ' biotonus ' (from the Greek βίος, life, and tonus) *i.e.* the tonus of the living cell. As regards the relationship A/D Verworn says that it is usually equal to 1, *i.e.* that assimilation and dissimilation balance one another, and that a change in one of these will always produce a corresponding change in the other.

I must, however, object to this definition of the term tonus, in that it does not correspond in the least to the well-established meaning of the word. That the tonus of the living cell and the Verwornian biotonus are two quite different things is obvious from the fact that when the function of the cell increases (which is shown in a muscle-cell by stronger contraction), this naturally comes from an increase of dissimilation accompanied by a corresponding increase of assimilation and the connection A/D remains = 1 ; *i.e.* there is an increase of the real tonus of the cell (a stronger contraction in the case of the muscle-cell) while its biotonus A/D according to Verworn remains the same = 1. It will be found on the whole that Verworn's biotonus of a cell, the relation between its assimilation and dissimilation, will remain unchanged, regardless of and uninfluenced by the extent to which the real tonus of the cell may have changed in one direction or the other ; therefore Verworn's biotonus cannot be identical with the real tonus of the cell.

That the fraction A/D does not and cannot express the tonus of the cell, is very obvious if we imagine an alteration in the relation between A and D, an alteration of their values. If, for example, we leave A unchanged and imagine that D is increased for a moment, the curious situation will arise that Verworn's biotonus of the cell will decrease for the fraction A/D will be less than 1, while the real tonus of the cell which depends entirely on the amount of dissimilation, will on the contrary increase. Similarly, if we imagine A to be raised while D remains unchanged, A/D will then be greater than 1, *i.e.* Verworn's biotonus of the cell will increase while its real tonus does not change as the dissimilation has not risen. From this we see clearly that the relation between assimilation and dissimilation in the cell cannot express its tonus, in the meaning that science has once and for all given to this word.

Verworn himself points out that, on the other hand, the relation between assimilation and dissimilation may be considered as an expression for the growth or disappearance of the cell, or for the amount of storage in the cell and for its use of reserve material, *i.e.* as that which is called the potential energy of the cell, an expression borrowed from chemistry. Verworn thinks that growth and tonus cannot be separated as no sharp dividing line can be drawn between them. In reality, however, they are two quite different phenomena, between which there may at times be direct opposition.

The preliminary condition for the growth of a cell or for its capability of storing reserve material is that its assimilation should exceed its dissimilation, that A/D should be greater than 1 ; but this does not necessarily involve a change in the actual tonus which depends only on the amount of dissimilation. A rise in the actual tonus which comes from an increase of dissimilation may on the contrary prevent both growth and storage if assimilation does not keep pace with dissimilation or (preferably) exceed it. Because a cell, for example, a muscle-cell, grows, its tonus does not necessarily increase ; and because the tonus of a muscle rises, the latter does not necessarily grow.

The name biotonus for the relation between assimilation and dissimilation cannot therefore be justified; this relation A/D is of comparatively little importance and may be regarded as an expression for the growth and disappearance of the cell or for the amount of its storage and its use of reserve material. I have already touched upon Verworn's biotonus theory because Lehmann, as we saw, tries to use it in support of his dynamic theory of feeling in its latest form ; and of course a hypothesis such as Lehmann's which has failed from the outset, is not improved by the support of Verworn's equally mistaken theory.

After having thus limited and determined the use of the term tonus and its meaning, we may proceed to apply the law of the tonus of all living organisms to the human brain.

Just as this law holds good for the cells of muscles and glands, it also applies to nerve- and brain-cells and to the centres and organs composed of these. The psycho-motor centres from which innervation goes to all transversely-striated muscles, have tonus ; as long as they are living and uninjured, they always show a certain degree of their specific function, motor innervation, which again is the chief reason why the muscles innervated by them are always (even when most in repose) to some extent contracted.

Carl Lange * was the first to draw attention to 'latent innervation' as he calls this phenomenon, the continuous flow of innervation from the psycho-motor centres to the muscles, which is indeed the expression for the tonus of these cells. The centres of the sense-organs and the higher intellectual centres which deal with their sensations and ideas must of course also have tonus.

The German psychiatrist, Griesinger, well known in his own time, was probably the first who emphasized the existence of intellectual tonus. He treats the question both in his Psychiatry (1871) and (especially) in a treatise on Psychic Reflex Actions which was used as an introduction to his posthumously published Collected Treatises (1872). In these works he maintains that in the brain there is always " a mean condition of apparent repose," " a tonus of the organ of ideation." Griesinger's demonstration of a ' psychic tonus ' (psychic being used here in the narrower meaning of the word in the sense of ' intellectual ') seems to have left hardly any trace in contemporary or in subsequent psychological research. At any rate psycho-physics and its heir, modern psycho - physiology, know nothing of it, although it might be thought that intellectual tonus was such a fundamental pheno-

* *Rygmarvens Pathologie*, Copenhagen, 1871–76.

menon that any psychological research which paid no attention to it, would necessarily be a complete failure.

This is not the case in empirical psychology which is much closer to life, especially in the form in which we find it in Höffding's works. When Höffding in his Psychology writes, " that every organic being, apart from outside influences, is completely ' spontaneous ' in a given function and that outside influences can produce only changes in this function and not anything quite new," this involves a recognition on the part of experimental psychology of the two main laws applied in this chapter to the activity of the brain and its centres, *i.e.* the laws of the specific energy and of the tonus of the living cell.

As I already mentioned in Chapter II, Höffding points out in accordance with the latter law, that our attitude towards those impressions from our environment which arouse our sensations is never passive or merely receptive. In fact, in order that a sensation may be produced, not only an outer impression is required, but also at the same time a certain readiness of the particular brain-centre, a turning towards the impression, a definite activity of the brain-cells, without which no sensation can arise. This activity, this readiness of the brain-cells which receive the sensation, is the phenomenon which physiology calls the tonus of the cells and psychology calls attention. Attention, is, however, the elementary form of will. There is only a difference of degree between the simple activity which appears in the functioning of sensations and ideas as attention, and the highest form of intellectual activity (will) which is seen in logical thought, in choice and determination; this is therefore also a psychic correlate of the tonus of the cells in question. Thought and will, as I have pointed out before, are not two different elementary mental phenomena but two sides or properties of the same psychic phenomenon, which correspond physiologically to the specific energy of the cells concerned or to their tonus.

As a logical consequence of the demonstration of intellectual and psycho-motor tonus by Griesinger and Lange, I have already in my earlier works * added to these a tonus of the feeling-centre; and I have shown that the assumption of a feeling - tonus not only agrees with the results of empirical psychology but is absolutely necessary to explain what life teaches us about the psychic element of feeling. In human life there is no moment without a certain feeling-tone, which corresponds to the tonus of the centre at that moment. In ordinary circumstances the feeling-tone may not be very prominent; but in this respect it is like the intellectual and

* Among others in a treatise published in 1904 on the Anatomical and Physiological Basis of Feeling.

EMOTION AND INSANITY

psycho-motor tonus, in fact, like the tonus of all other organs. The tonus of other organs is also not very obvious in their mean function ; only when it changes in a positive or negative direction is attention directed more definitely to it. The fact that a feeling or idea has a pleasure- or a displeasure-tone, means that the corresponding physiological process produces an increase or a decrease in the function of certain cells in the feeling-centre which is recognized psychically as pleasure or displeasure. When this increase or decrease in function affects the majority of the cells in the feeling-centre or the whole centre, this means that the particular intellectual process with its pleasure- or displeasure-tone, has caused the genesis of a feeling, a mood or an emotion of an exalted or a depressed nature, by which the feeling-tone of simultaneous or immediately following processes is influenced and partly determined. And by the quantitative changes which appear at the same time in the intellectual and the psycho-motor region and follow the changes in the feeling-element, as well as by the suddenness, intensity and duration with which all this happens, the whole character of the feeling-state is determined as mood, emotion or feeling, as grief, anxiety or joy.

As I have already said, the feeling-centre must cover a considerable area and must be composed of a large number of brain-cells.

This is the necessary condition of the fact
that at the same moment there may be in
one part of the cells an increased activity
corresponding to pleasure while in another
part there may be a depressed function
corresponding to displeasure. In this way
the conditions arise which bring about that
group of feeling-states which I placed in the
second or higher order in the previous chapter,
and which are characterized psychologically
by the simultaneous presence of pleasure
and displeasure, and by different degrees of
these.

From this chapter then we see that by
looking at the human brain and its function
from a physiological point of view and by
applying to it definite physiological laws and
maxims, we may arrive at results which are
in exact agreement with empirical psychology, especially in the form given to it by
Höffding. It will be obvious that by this
means it is possible, to use my previous
phrase, to interpret psychology physiologically.
In reality the theory developed in this work
concerning the physiological activity of the
living organism of the brain is almost completely parallel with Höffding's account of
the corresponding psychic phenomena. Only
in one point I find it necessary to correct the
anatomy, physiology and pathology of psychology, and to alter the dividing line between

the intellectual side of mental life and the side which expresses itself in action.

The three psychic elements of empirical psychology, all of which are found with varying intensity and preponderance in every psychic process, correspond to three different brain-centres, the intellectual, the psychomotor and the emotional, each composed of its own special type of cells. This is the law of the specific energy of the cell as applied to the brain.

The psychological observation that in every psychic process elements of all three types are contained in a greater or less degree, corresponds to the physiological fact that brain-centres, like all other organs composed of living cells, are always functioning to some extent. This is the law of the tonus of all living organs as applied to the brain.

The observation founded on a psychological analysis of the mental diseases of mood and the corresponding normal states of feeling, that all these differ from one another only quantitatively, corresponds to the fundamental physiological law that the living cell under physiological (and certain pathological) conditions can change in intensity only with an increase or decrease of its specific function.

INDEX

INDEX

Mania. (See also *Manic-depressive Psychosis*), 45 ff.
Manic-depressive Psychosis, 34, Chap. III., *passim*
—— complex types, 49 ff.
Melancholia. (See also *Manic-depressive Psychosis*), 46 ff.
Mental diseases. (See *Manic-depressive Psychosis*.)
Mind-body problem, 90 f.
Mood, Disorders of. (See *Manic-depressive Psychosis*.)
Moods. (See *Affective States*.)

Nerve-tracts, 9, 111
Neurone, 93, 94, 96
Niessl-Mayendorf, 107
Normal mental conditions, explained by study of abnormal conditions, 9, 10, 41 ff., 48, 51, 55, 61, 65, 107, 126

Pain, 23 ff.
Passions, 69 ff.
Pathology, cerebral, 9, 33
—— Neuro-, 9
—— (See also *Psycho-pathology*.)
Phrenology, 114 ff.
Physiology, 3 ff., 33, 34, 77, Chap. IV., *passim*.
Pleasure, 16, 17, 46 ff., Chap. IV., *passim*
Primitive peoples, 40, 71
Psychiatrists, 8 ff., 42, 121
Psychiatry, 7, 34, Chap. III., *passim*, 89, 112
Psychologists, 5, 7, 10, 107
Psychology, 4 ff., Chaps. II. and III., *passim*, 89, 104, 125 ; empirical, 11, 15, 115, 122, 123, 125 f.

Psycho-motor factors. (See *Activity, Centre, Inhibition, Innervation*.)
Psycho-pathology. (See *Psychiatry*.)
Psycho-physics, 5, 121
Psycho-physiology, 6, 7, 11, 116, 121
Psychoses. (See *Manic-depressive*.)

Self-control, 40, 44
Sensation, 20, 22 ff., 26 32, 33, 97 ff., 105, 108, 110 ff., 122
Smell, 100, 101, 103
Sound, 98, 101
Specific Energy (of living cell), 19, 76, 91, 122, 126
Speech, lack of clearness in daily, 22 ff., 45, 52, 60, 65, 74, 78 ff.
—— (See also *Centre*.)
Stupor, 52

Taste, 100, 101, 109
Thalbitzer, 107, 109
Thought, 26 ff., 34, 75, 123
Tigerstedt, 23, 111
Tonus, 29, 116 ff., 126

Unpleasure. (See *Displeasure*.)

Verworn, 29, 96, 117 ff.

Weygandt, 49, 55
Will, 15, 28 ff., 31-35, 123
Wundt (Wilhelm), 18 ff., 35